SALVESTROLS
JOURNEYS TO WELLNESS

Copyright © 2013 Clinical Intelligence Corp.
All rights reserved.

No part of this publication may be reproduced,
stored in a retrieval system, or transmitted in any form or by
any means, electronic, mechanical, photocopying, recording,
or otherwise, for any purpose, without the written prior
permission of the author.

Salvestrol® is a registered trademark of
Salvestrol Natural Products Ltd.

ISBN 978-1494395780

Typeset at SpicaBookDesign in Plantin

Published in Canada.

Dedicated to all of the cancer patients that I have had the privilege of meeting over the years. May your strength, humour, compassion and humanity serve as an inspiration to us all.

DISCLAIMER

The intent of this book is to provide an introduction to the personal experiences that many have had using Salvestrols to manage their disease.

This book is not intended as a medical or nutritional reference. Neither is it intended as a definitive source of information about Salvestrols. People requiring expert assistance in medical or nutritional matters should consult a professional. This book should not be used in the diagnosis of any medical condition.

Every effort has been made to provide complete, accurate and timely information. However, there may be mistakes both typographical and in content. The reader is well advised to use this book as a general guide from which they can conduct their own research.

The author and copyright holder shall have neither liability nor responsibility to any entity or person with respect to any loss or damage caused, or alleged to be caused, directly or indirectly by the concepts or information contained in this book.

PREFACE

I still remember the first time someone in my life was diagnosed with cancer. Well, actually my grandmother was the first but at the age of five I was not really aware of what was going on other than that grandma went to the hospital and never came back. Quite a few decades later I was out of the office at a business meeting, came back and was told that a friend and former colleague had stopped by the office and was very insistent that he needed to see me. As it turned out he had been diagnosed with cancer. It was such a shock that I can't even remember which cancer he had. Unfortunately I was unable to see him prior to his admission to hospital. Apparently the cancer was very advanced by the time he was diagnosed. I headed up to the hospital to see him filled with trepidation. What do you say to your friend that is now admitted to hospital with life threatening cancer? He had four children at home! What will he be like? What will he look like? What if his family is there? What will I say to them? How can I possibly help with this?

I got to the hospital and paced around the parking lot, chain smoking (now there's a winning strategy when you are about to visit your friend with cancer eh?) while pondering these questions. I came up with no answers but soon decided that pacing around the parking lot was not doing anyone any good. I found his room. My friend was lying there with the head of the bed raised to help him breathe better. He gave me his usual mischievous grin and said 'hi'. What the hell? He was the same as he ever was! I sat down and we started to chat as we usually did. He was heavily medicated for pain and began slipping in and out of consciousness. He knew about his situation and it was not good. He had always been fun to spend time with, sometimes too much fun but we won't go into that here. In speaking with him it struck me that although his life would soon be over he wanted to make sure that he filled his remaining moments with the normalcy of interactions with family and friends and surprisingly he maintained his sense of humour – even about his impending death!

He didn't last long – only a few days. I managed to see him only a couple of times but he taught me a lot in those brief encounters. Through his example he pointed out that even as we face death, it is our relationships that sustain us. Throughout life this never changes. There is no magic phrase, speech or saying that we can use to make everything right in these circumstances, there is only love, friendship, compassion and perhaps a little humour.

Little did I know at the time that my encounters with people diagnosed with cancer would start to escalate and come much closer to home. My father was diagnosed, his brother was diagnosed, friends of the family were diagnosed, in-laws were diagnosed,

PREFACE

my mother was diagnosed. My small family attended twelve funerals in three years. It got so that no one in our house wanted to answer the phone.

During this time I met a small group of cancer researchers in the UK. I was intrigued by the work they were doing. I had come across some of their research papers and wanted to learn more. One evening, while in London on business I decided to phone the laboratory of one of these researchers. After reading about their work I had decided that these were the sort of individuals that did not keep bankers hours – they were likely still in the lab. The phone rang and just as expected one of the researchers picked up the phone – Prof. Gerry Potter. We had a very interesting chat about his work, exchanged email addresses and began an email dialogue. We got together on a subsequent trip to the UK and began talking about how we could work together. We have been working together ever since and consequently I have now met a huge number of people that have been diagnosed with cancer.

To state the obvious, a cancer diagnosis is extremely difficult for most people. Yet, I meet person after person who work through this challenge with strength, grace, humour and compassion. The cancer sufferers that I have met have been truly inspirational. There have been so many occasions during which I have met someone with a serious cancer situation who upon seeing me expresses concern for me because I happen to have a runny nose at the time or I have hit my finger with a hammer or some other minor malady! It is as if their own situation has heightened their compassion for others. All I can say is that if you are losing faith in humanity you probably haven't met anyone who is dealing with cancer lately because those that I meet would restore your faith in humanity and leave you humbled by the interaction.

Throughout this time I have had occasion to make many new friends and have had occasion to work with some to record their progress from diagnosis to recovery. In doing this work the intent was to make this information available to practitioners. Consequently many of the experiences described in this book have a version that has appeared in the Journal of Orthomolecular Medicine or the International Journal of Phytotherapy. Recording these successful outcomes has been enormously rewarding. These experiences have been expanded here to bring them up to date (that is, up to February 2013), to include information that wasn't included originally when new information has become available and to make them more widely accessible. These experiences are presented here in the hope that people will be able to take advantage of the experiences of others to assist with the choices that need to be made for their own cancer or the cancer of their patients.

Do these experiences include the magic bullet that will see all cancer sufferers fully recover? No. At this point no such magic bullet exists. With that said they do point to strategies that brought these people through to renewed good health so it is well worth the effort of investigating these strategies for future situations because they may represent the strategy that will bring about the desired outcome.

ACKNOWLEDGEMENTS

I owe a great debt of gratitude to all of those that have shared their stories that are re-told here. The road from diagnosis to recovery is often filled with fear, anguish and best left in the past and yet these individuals have contributed their time and shared their experiences and medical facts so that others may benefit. Thank you all very much. It has been a great pleasure working with each of you. May your futures be filled with organic fruit and vegetables!

I also owe a great deal of thanks to Roxanne Brass whose comment 'just read the stories' served as the inspiration for writing this book. The comment was made to her husband while he was reading my previous book and when I heard it I knew she was absolutely right – it is the stories that we really want to hear. Thanks Roxanne for that dose of reality.

Of course great thanks are due to the research team, Anthony Daniels, Dan Burke, Gerry Potter and Robbie Wood for filling serious work with moments of hilarity, the fuel that drives it all! And of course great thanks are due to the entire crew: Luke Daniels; Andy O'Keefe; Toni Wright; Lucy Fazackerley; Ian Morrison; Cassandra Miller; Dave and Maureen Vousden; Gary Gwynne; Kevin Coyne; Vanessa Ascencao; Darragh Hammond; Dominic Galvin; Tommy & Irene Kobberskov; Bolke Koster; Aart-Jan Breet; Dick den Hartog; Gerard Alserda; Edward Winfield; and Manuel Pozo – your spirit of collaboration and cooperation serves us all.

Special thanks to Dr. Michael Schachter and Jacquie Beattie for their very detailed and thorough review of this book and for their many helpful suggestions. This book is vastly improved as a result of their efforts.

Great thanks to Robbie Wood, Ian Morrison, Luke Daniels, Kay Butler, Frances Fuller, Anthony Daniels, Dave Vousden and Gary Gwynne for their valuable comments on the early drafts of this book.

Many thanks to Iryna Spica, the book designer, who has turned my manuscripts into books. Iryna has designed this book and my previous book (English, Spanish and German versions) and done a magnificent job. Iryna approaches her work with skill, enthusiasm and cheerfulness and is a complete pleasure to work with.

Thank you to the Journal of Orthomolecular Medicine and the International Journal of Phytotherapy for publishing the original case study articles and thank you for your permission to re-tell these stories here.

Thank you to Health Action Network Society for their permission to re-tell the 'Final Story' here.

Great thanks to Bev, Meg and Sam for your sustaining level of support, encouragement and input through all my endeavours.

> *The beauty of Salvestrols is that you don't need to paddle up the Amazon to find them – if you grow organically you can find them in your own garden regardless of where you live.*
>
> Public lecture,
> New Zealand, February 2013

CONTENTS

1	**Introduction**	1
	Chapter notes	11
2	**Bladder cancer**	14
	Papillary urothelial carcinoma, kidney cancer and pancreatic cancer	15
	Recurrent, non-muscle invasive bladder cancer	21
	Chapter notes	25
3	**Breast cancer**	27
	Breast cancer, stage 1	28
	Breast cancer, stage 3	31
	Breast cancer, aggressive stage 3	35
	Chapter notes	40
4	**Colorectal Cancer**	41
	Possible Colon Cancer – no biopsy done	42
	Squamous Cell Carcinoma of the Anus	45
	Chapter notes	48

5	**Chronic Lymphocytic Leukaemia**	**50**
	Chronic Lymphocytic Leukaemia	52
	Chapter notes	56
6	**Hodgkin Lymphoma** **(also known as Hodgkin's disease)**	**57**
	Hodgkin Lymphoma, stage 3B	59
	Chapter notes	62
7	**Primary Liver Cancer**	**63**
	Liver Cancer – stage 2	64
	Chapter notes	68
8	**Primary lung Cancer**	**69**
	Squamous-cell carcinoma of the lung – stage 2-3	70
	Chapter notes	75
9	**Melanoma**	**76**
	Melanoma – stage 4	77
	Chapter notes	81
10	**Peritoneal Cancer with Metastases in the Ovaries**	**82**
	Primary Peritoneal Carcinoma – stage 3	83
	Chapter notes	89

11 Prostate Cancer — 91

Prostate Cancer — 92

Prostate Cancer — 96

Prostate Cancer, Gleason Score 6 (3+3) — 98

Chapter notes — 102

12 Benign Prostatic Hyperplasia — 103

Benign Prostatic Hyperplasia — 104

Chapter notes — 107

13 Study Follow Up — 108

Study Overview — 109

Rapid Responders — 111

Low Salvestrol Intake Responders — 112

Rapid Response at Low Daily Salvestrol Intake — 113

Remission Follow Up — 114

Length of Time in Remission — 117

What About Those That Respond Very Slowly? — 121

What Did We Learn From the Follow Up? — 126

14 When are We Well? — 128

Ovarian Cancer, Stage 3 — 128

15 One Last Story	**135**
16 The Need for Better Diagnostics	**138**
Metabolite Test	142
Proteomic Test	145
Summary	147
17 Conclusion	**149**
Glossary	157
References in the popular press	162
Bibliography	171
Index	183
For more information	190
The Author	192
Clinical Intelligence Publishing	193

SALVESTROLS
JOURNEYS TO WELLNESS

1.
INTRODUCTION

Eat your vegetables! We have all heard this before and likely from our mothers. Good advice, but when my mother told me to eat my vegetables, the directive came without explanation, and I was smart enough not to ask for one. We are told that we should increase our consumption of fruits and vegetables, but when we ask why, we rarely get a satisfactory answer. We will typically get an answer such as, 'studies of people who have a diet made up of abundant fruits and vegetables enjoy greater health benefits and reduced risk of cancer'. This doesn't really tell us how this works – after all it may be the case that people that eat more fruit and vegetables also take more exercise – we don't know.

About a decade ago I came across the work of a group of English cancer researchers that provided a real explanation of how this works – a mechanism that explained how eating fruits and vegetables would not just prevent cancer but could kill cancer. The group consisted of Prof. Gerry Potter, Prof. Dan Burke and Anthony Daniels. Gerry is a medicinal chemist, Dan is a pharmacologist/toxicologist and Anthony is an engineer.

In the early 1990s these men were conducting work that would facilitate their later collaboration on explaining the link between fruit and vegetable consumption and cancer.

Gerry was working at The Institute of Cancer Research in London. The team that he was involved with was interested in prostate cancer, and in particular, the role of testosterone in prostate cancer progression. They were interested in developing methods of reducing testosterone production in the hopes of slowing prostate cancer growth. To this end they knew that an enzyme, CYP17 (pronounced 'sip 17'), was instrumental in the pathway for production of androgens such as testosterone. Gerry has a fantastic ability to visualise complex chemical and biochemical shapes. He began working with CYP17 and designed a compound that would inhibit the operation of this enzyme and consequently the production of testosterone. The compound that he designed was Abiraterone acetate, now known by the trade name Zytiga®. This medication was approved by the United States Food and Drug Administration for the treatment of advanced prostate cancer in June 2012, 22 years after Gerry developed it.

This compound worked in a very different way than typical cancer therapies. It was not toxicity to

INTRODUCTION

human cells that brought about the benefit, it was the combination of Abiraterone acetate and CYP17 which resulted in CYP17 being switched off, resulting in less testosterone production that brought about the benefit. This made it a highly targeted therapy and the subsequent testing proved that this was a very effective approach, especially for end stage prostate cancer sufferers[1, 2, 3]. This work on Abiraterone followed from the preference in prostate cancer therapeutics to come up with therapies that would lower the levels of testosterone or androgens in the body as testosterone tends to stimulate prostate cancer growth. Gerry received his third award from the Royal Society of Chemistry for his design of this drug. He is the only scientist to ever receive more than one of these awards[4].

While Gerry was working on development of targeted cancer therapies in London, Dan Burke and his students were investigating another CYP enzyme at the Medical School in Aberdeen. The enzyme was CYP1B1 (pronounced 'sip one be one'). They initially discovered that CYP1B1 showed up in soft tissue sarcomas but did not show up in the surrounding healthy tissue[5]. The finding was interesting but did not cause too much of a stir. Dan and his students were intrigued and decided to investigate other cancers. They found the same result in breast cancer[6, 7], namely that CYP1B1 was present in the breast cancer cells, but not in the surrounding normal breast cells. They then moved on to investigate a broad array of cancers and found the same result of CYP1B1 being present in cancer cells of the colon, lung, oesophagus, skin, lymph nodes, brain, and testis, with no detectable presence in the surrounding healthy tissue[8, 9]. This cumulative body of evidence was very exciting as it indicated that CYP1B1 might serve as a universal cancer marker, and as such, could be used both as a target for cancer therapy and as a target to use for diagnostic purposes. In short, CYP1B1 could be the Holy Grail of cancer research. At this point, laboratories around the world started investigating CYP1B1 and it is now widely regarded as a universal cancer marker of great utility because it shows up in the various cancers but is absent from healthy tissue.

Meanwhile Anthony was working on developing methods of reliably extracting natural compounds from plant materials and investigating the utility of botanical compounds for real world applications in health, agriculture and environmental remediation. He became particularly adept at extracting compounds from herbs and foods – something that was about to become very important for the advancement of cancer research. As an example, he developed a botanical extract for the preservation of bananas during shipping to market to reduce the health consequences of the synthetic compounds that were in use. Most recently, he has developed a machine that uses botanical extracts for environmental remediation. There are enormous opportunities for this type of remediation that can return land to productive use.

Dan Burke left Aberdeen and took an academic post as head of the School of Pharmacy in Leicester. He then recruited Gerry Potter to his department at

INTRODUCTION

the University to develop a prodrug for CYP1B1. Dan discussed his work on CYP1B1 with Gerry and outlined the problem that needed to be solved. Following on his success with Abiraterone for CYP17, Gerry set to work on CYP1B1 and designed a prodrug for it. The drug was designed to be activated through metabolism by CYP1B1 to produce a metabolite that would initiate apoptosis (programmed cell death) in the cancer cell. In this way, the drug would be absolutely targeted to the cancer and leave little room for harmful side effects. The drug, Stilserene, worked exceptionally well in laboratory tests on a wide array of cancers, including those known to be chemotherapy resistant. As Gerry likes to point out with a grin on his face, the object was to have patients that were "still serene while undergoing cancer treatment"! Stilserene was patented and started its painfully slow passage through the clinical trial process.

Throughout this drug development process, many discussions were held as to why CYP1B1 would be present in cancer cells and not in healthy tissue – what was its function? The professors hypothesised that CYP1B1 must be a rescue mechanism for ridding the body of aberrant cancer cells. Enzymes work by changing the shape, structure, and often function of compounds that can bind with them. If this hypothesis were true, then a prediction that could be derived was that the compounds for CYP1B1 to metabolise would come from one's diet. Dan and Gerry began to re-examine the structure of the prodrug Stilserene and realised that they had seen similar compounds in plant biology. They began a search for plant compounds that could be metabolised by CYP1B1 to see if they would have the same anti-cancer property as their prodrug. They found some! Tests were performed and indeed these natural compounds performed in the same way that the prodrug Stilserene performed its function, that is, selective targeting of CYP1B1 and consequent destruction of the cancer cell. These dietary compounds were metabolised by CYP1B1 and the metabolite brought about the destruction of the cancerous cell[10, 11, 12]. These natural compounds were named Salvestrols.

These natural Salvestrols have the same targeted, prodrug, selectivity as the synthetic drug Stilserene. Nature has had a lot more time to work this out than Gerry, and he found that nature produced some Salvestrols with much higher selectivity than Stilserene. By selectivity we mean that the metabolite produced by CYP1B1 was able to kill cancer cells because of the presence of CYP1B1, but not kill normal cells, which contained no CYP1B1 and hence no metabolite.

Here was a specific, tested mechanism to explain how certain dietary compounds could prevent and treat cancer. We ingest Salvestrols from organic fruit and vegetables. They are absorbed and transported through the body. When they encounter the CYP1B1 enzyme in cancer cells the CYP1B1 enzyme metabolises these Salvestrols, producing a metabolite that induces the death of the cancer cell. It is a very elegant mechanism and it provides great credibility to the hypothesis that CYP1B1 is a rescue enzyme. It

INTRODUCTION

also indicates that cancer can be viewed as a dietary deficiency. When the diet is deficient in Salvestrols, cancer cells can proliferate. When a diet is rich in Salvestrols, this rescue mechanism maintains good health of the body. If the body has cancer cells, the ingestion of Salvestrols tends to get rid of the cancer cells and returns the body to good health.

With the discovery of Salvestrols came the question of how to make this knowledge available to people that were suffering with cancer. The initial approach was to put together a diet to highlight the foods that would deliver Salvestrols. Gerry produced what is known as the Green and Red diet. He also got in touch with Anthony Daniels to discuss whether or not it would be possible to formulate a supplement to provide the higher levels of daily intake that people would likely need if they were diagnosed with cancer.

Early on it was known that a variety of herbs were good sources of Salvestrols, but Anthony knew that changes to the regulatory framework for health products made extraction from herbs a problematic direction to take. A program of work was initiated to screen fruits and vegetables for Salvestrols, and it produced some very interesting findings. In short, it showed that fruits and vegetables that were grown using traditional or organic methods produced significantly higher quantities of Salvestrols than those grown conventionally. Furthermore, they found that heritage varieties (plants that have not been bred or modified to change their original characteristics) produced vastly higher quantities of Salvestrols. Why?

Salvestrols are part of the plants defence against predation, particularly against fungal attack, and they are produced in response to predation. Consequently if a plant is sprayed with agents that reduce predation, or reduce fungal attacks, the plant does not produce Salvestrols. This is why these beneficial compounds are not part of our typical diet. Furthermore, plants have been bred to produce sweeter fruits and vegetables in an attempt to increase their market appeal. Salvestrols typically have a bitter taste and therefore they don't contribute to the notion of a highly marketable fruit or vegetable. This is why when we look at the levels of Salvestrols in heritage crops they are vastly higher than those found in modern varieties[13, 14].

This has been a very brief introduction to Salvestrols. A more in depth discussion of the research and development of Salvestrols is provided in my first book "Salvestrols – Nature's Defence Against Cancer".

Here is the summary:

- Salvestrols are most abundant in organically grown fruits and vegetables especially heritage varieties.
- CYP1B1 is a universal cancer marker that shows up in all the various cancers but not in healthy tissue.
- Salvestrols are food based compounds that when metabolised by CYP1B1, produce a metabolite that induces apoptosis in the cancer cell.

INTRODUCTION

- Salvestrols are part of the plants defence mechanism against predation such as fungal attack.
- In the presence of a large dietary source of Salvestrols such as from organically grown heritage crops, this mechanism works to maintain good health by killing off aberrant cells. In dietary deficiencies in which Salvestrol ingestion is chronically low, aberrant cells proliferate. By addressing this dietary deficiency, the mechanism can return the body to good health.

Since the discovery of Salvestrols, many people have adopted dietary change and Salvestrol supplementation as a means of addressing their dietary deficiency after receiving a diagnosis of cancer. We have had the opportunity to work closely with a number of these individuals to study their journey from diagnosis to recovery. These studies cover a wide cross section of cancers: anal; bladder; breast; colon; leukaemia; liver; lung; lymphoma; melanoma; peritoneal; and prostate. They represent the situations of people from a number of different countries: Canada; England; Korea; New Zealand; South Africa; and the United States. Obviously both males and females are involved and they represent a cross-section of ages from 36 to 94.

Over the last year, up until February 2013, I have been conducting a follow up on these people to determine how they have got on after achieving remission. The first eleven chapters document each of their situations as they worked through to remission. I then go through the data obtained through the follow up to highlight the lessons learned. From the lessons learned I introduce two situations that challenge our thinking about cancer and cancer progression. The individuals that are documented leave us with food for thought. Finally I introduce the work that we are conducting on the development of blood tests for early cancer detection, disease monitoring and determination of treatment efficacy as these tests will alleviate a great deal of the uncertainty that accompanies many people's journey from diagnosis to recovery.

To better understand the chapters that follow I need to give a brief explanation of Salvestrol points. When we take pills or capsules we are used to seeing the amount of a drug or nutrient given in a unit such as milligrams or international units. This follows from a pharmaceutical model where a single active agent is being given. Salvestrols are derived from food and they constitute a class of compounds rather than a single compound. Each unique Salvestrol compound has its own characteristic selectivity. This fact makes it unreasonable to indicate amount in milligrams, as the potency of the product would vary greatly depending on which mix of Salvestrols were used. Salvestrol points have been developed as a metric of potency that can be used with any mixture of Salvestrols. Capsules are produced that contain 100 points, 350 points, 1,000 points and 2,000 points. After reviewing the pharmacokinetics of these various Salvestrol compounds, our best estimate is that an intake of 4,000

INTRODUCTION

to 6,000 Salvestrol points per day would likely be required to overcome a long term dietary deficiency that had resulted in a cancer diagnosis. However, much higher doses have been used with cancers of the brain and in advanced metastatic disease. Once remission has been achieved it is thought that a daily intake of 2,000 Salvestrol points per day should be sufficient to maintain good health.

The situations described here are meant to show how this Salvestrol/CYP1B1 rescue mechanism can assist some of those afflicted with cancer in their return to good health. They are not meant to convey a sense that these are the outcomes that everyone should expect. Certainly people have made dietary change and utilised Salvestrol supplementation without achieving remission. Many factors contribute to the success or failure in individual cases, including dietary choices, exercise level, psychosocial stresses, type and amount of conventional therapies and exposures to toxins in the environment.

CHAPTER NOTES:

1. Attard G, Belldegrun AS, de Bono JS (2005). Selective blockade of androgenic steroid synthesis by novel lyase inhibitors as a therapeutic strategy for treating metastatic prostate cancer. *BJU Int.* **96** (9): 1241–6.
2. Attard G, Reid AHM, Yap TA, Raynaud F, Dowsett M, Settatree S, Barrett M, Parker C, Martins V, Folkerd E, Clark J, Cooper CS, Kaye SB, Dearnaley D, Lee G, de Bono JS (2008). Phase I Clinical Trial of a Selective

Inhibitor of CYP17, Abiraterone Acetate, Confirms That Castration-Resistant Prostate Cancer Commonly Remains Hormone Driven. *Journal of Clinical Oncology* : 4563.

3. Attard G, Reid A, A'Hern R, Parker C, Oommen N, Folkerd E, Messiou C, Molife L, Maier G, Thompson E, Olmos D, Sinha R, Lee G, Dowsett M, Kaye S, Dearnaley D, Kheoh T, Molina A, and de Bono J (2009). Selective Inhibition of CYP17 With Abiraterone Acetate Is Highly Active in the Treatment of Castration-Resistant Prostate Cancer. *Journal of Clinical Oncology*, (23):3742-8.

4. Schaefer BA. December 2012. *Gerry Potter Honoured for his Development of Abiraterone Acetone,* www.helping-HANS.org.

5. Murray GI, McKay JA, Weaver RJ, et al, (1993) Cytochrome P450 expression is a common molecular event in soft tissue sarcomas. *Journal of Pathology*, :49–52,

6. McKay J, Melvin W, Ahsee A, Ewen S, Greenlee W, Marcus C, Burke M, Murray G (1995) Expression Of Cytochrome-P450 Cyp1b1 In Breast-Cancer *FEBS Letters* (2): 270-272.

7. McFadyen MCE, Breeman S, Payne S, et al. Immunohistochemical localization of cytochrome P450 CYP1B1 in breast cancer with monoclonal antibodies specific for CYP1B1. *Journal of Histochemistry and Cytochemistry,* 1999; :1457–64.

8. Murray GI, Taylor MC, McFadyen MCE, McKay JA, Greenlee WF, Burke MD, Melvin WT (1997) Tumor specific expression of cytochrome P450 CYP 1B1. *Cancer Research*: 3026-3031.

INTRODUCTION

9. Murray GI, Melvin WT, Greenlee WF, Burke MD, (2001) Regulation, function, and tissue-specific expression of cytochrome P450 CYP1B1. *Annual Review of Pharmacology and Toxicology*: 297-316.

10. Potter GA (2002) The role of CYP 1B1 as a tumour suppressor enzyme. *British Journal of Cancer,* (Suppl 1), S12, 2002.

11. Potter GA, Burke DM (2006) Salvestrols – Natural Products with Tumour Selective Activity. *Journal of Orthomolecular Medicine*, 21, : 34-36.

12. Salvestrols ... Natural Plant and Cancer Agents? *British Naturopathic Journal,* :1,10-13.

13. Li NC, & Wakeman M. (October 2009) High-performance liquid chromatography comparison of eight beneficial secondary plant metabolites in the flesh and peel or 15 varieties of apples. *The Pharmaceutical Journal*, supplement Vol. , B40.

14. Li NC, & Wakeman M. (2009) High-performance liquid chromatography comparison of eight beneficial secondary plant metabolites in the flesh and peel or 15 varieties of apples. *Journal of Pharmacy and Pharmacology*, supplement , A132.

2.
BLADDER CANCER

Bladder cancer usually starts in the cells lining the inside of the bladder – the transitional cells. Bladder cancer is among the top 10 most commonly diagnosed cancers in New Zealand and the incidence is approximately three times higher in males than females. According to the New Zealand Health Information Service there were 407 new cases of bladder cancer diagnosed in males during the year 2000 representing 4.3% of all new cancer diagnoses for males. There were 169 new cases of bladder cancer diagnosed in females, which represented 2.0% of all new cancer diagnoses for females.[1] This situation is comparable to that found in the United Kingdom. In 2008, UK bladder cancer diagnoses constituted 3.2% of new cancer diagnoses with about five bladder cancer diagnoses in men for every two bladder cancer diagnoses in women.[2]

Bladder cancer usually presents initially with blood in the urine. Smoking and occupational exposure to carcinogens are the two most common risk factors for the development of bladder cancer. Bladder cancers have a high rate of recurrence[3] and are typically treated with a bladder sparing transurethral resection of the bladder cancer (surgical removal of the cancer which is carried out by entering the bladder through the urethra, the tube through which urine passes).[4] In England and Wales men who have had a bladder cancer diagnosis have a 57% chance of being alive five years after the initial diagnosis. For women the five-year survival is even less at 47%.[5]

PAPILLARY UROTHELIAL CARCINOMA, KIDNEY CANCER AND PANCREATIC CANCER[6]

Date of diagnosis:	*May, 2010*
Age at diagnosis:	*62*
Sex:	*male*
Country of residence:	*New Zealand*
Salvestrol points per day:	*4,000 points*
Time from start of Salvestrol use to being told he was cancer free:	*6 months*
Time in remission with no evidence of cancer:	*16 months*

A 61-year-old man returned home from a business meeting and discovered blood in his urine. Having been involved in some heavy lifting on the previous day, he ascribed the incident to having strained something. The bleeding continued for two days and he then decided to visit his doctor. He told his doctor about the persistent blood in his urine for the previous three days (termed macroscopic haematuria). He also complained of swollen ankles and fungal infections on his nails (onychomycosis with concurrent paronychia). He was a non-smoker and had enjoyed good health except for a bout of septicaemia (infection in the bloodstream) following a knee operation eighteen years earlier. The doctor suspected an infection, took a urine sample, prescribed an antibiotic and referred him for an ultrasound. An ultrasound was performed two weeks later revealing an abnormal thickening near the left vesico-urethral junction (the junction between the bladder and the urethra, the tube through which urine passes from the bladder to the outside). He was referred for a flexible cystoscopy (a procedure during which the urologist is able to visualise the inside of the bladder using an instrument known as a cystoscope). The swollen ankles and fungal infections on his nails were deemed unimportant at the time.

Seven months elapsed before his appointment for flexible cystoscopy. The flexible cystoscopy found a small papillary tumour near the bladder neck close to the left vesico-urethral junction. An enlarged prostate was also noted and he was referred for surgery.

Two months later he was admitted for surgery. A transurethral resection of bladder tumour (TURBT) was performed. The surgery revealed a 2 cm papillary growth at the bladder neck and overlying left ureteric orifice (Note that tubes known as ureters connect the two kidneys with the bladder while the urethra is the tube that connects the bladder with the outside through which one urinates. The bladder neck is the area of the bladder adjacent to the connection with the urethra). No obvious disease was found in the ureter. A single dose of the chemotherapy drug epirubicin was instilled into the bladder.

Paracetamol (Panadol tablets) 500 mg, twice daily along with tramadol hydrochloride, 50 mg capsules, 1-2 daily, were recommended for pain relief but declined. Sodium citrotartrate (Ural) granules, 1 sachet daily, was also prescribed to reduce any burning sensation while passing urine – these were taken for two days following surgery. During surgery the urologist discovered that the tumour also involved part of the urethra and lesions were found on one of the kidneys. The urologist felt that the cancer had been removed from the bladder and urethra but the lesions on the kidney were not removed. The urologist was concerned about the possible return of the bladder cancer as he was well aware of the high rate of recurrence of bladder cancers.[2] The swelling in his ankles resolved quickly post-surgery. The urologist did not discuss the cause of this swelling with him.

Following surgery, the pathology report indicated that a grey/brown tumour, 20 mm x 17 mm in aggregate had been received and the histology report revealed a low grade papillary urothelial carcinoma with no invasion present. On the basis of this report he was referred to an oncologist. The oncologist indicated that the tumour had been a fast growing tumour that was quite rare. This opinion appeared to be at odds with the previously mentioned pathology report which had indicated that the tumour was a slow-growing low grade tumour. It was larger than they had anticipated from the prior flexible cystoscopy examination. An ultrasound and magnetic resonance imaging (MRI) were scheduled as part of a post-surgery, follow-up.

Seven months following the bladder surgery an ultrasound of the abdomen and pelvis was done and showed a tumour on the pancreas. An MRI was performed six weeks later and revealed a 4 cm tumour on the tail of the pancreas. No biopsies were taken as it was hospital policy to only perform a biopsy if the tumour had increased in size between successive images. This is an unfortunate policy since tumours of the pancreas can occasionally be benign and there are two types of pancreatic cancer. The more common adenocarcinoma of the pancreas has a very poor prognosis and the survival time from diagnosis is often six months to a year. The other cancer of the pancreas is a neuroendocrine cancer and the prognosis is better than that of the adenocarcinoma, with patients frequently surviving a few years following the diagnosis. One blood test frequently done in North America is the CA19-9. It is often elevated with the first type of cancer (the adenocarcinoma of the pancreas) but this test is not as commonly used in New Zealand and was not used in this situation. With the information that was available to the oncologist, who apparently assumed that the tumour of the pancreas was an adenocarcinoma, he informed this man that he had a life expectancy between 10 and 20 weeks. This individual was familiar with pancreatic adenocarcinomas and was well aware of the poor prognosis, especially when the tumour was located on the tail of the pancreas[7], as he had been active in fund raising for pancreatic cancer research. Consequently he was filled with fear.

Prior to his appointment for the ultrasound procedure that was done following his bladder cancer surgery, a former colleague had been in touch with him and upon hearing that he had been diagnosed with bladder cancer, suggested that he supplement his diet with Salvestrols. On three separate occasions his colleague made this recommendation and his suggestion was declined each time. Two weeks following the diagnosis of pancreatic cancer he agreed and commenced daily Salvestrol supplementation comprising two Salvestrol (2,000 point) capsules for a total daily intake of 4,000 Salvestrol points. This was added to his daily routine of 500 mg of vitamin C, a fish oil capsule, and an evening primrose capsule. No other changes to diet and lifestyle were made at this time, although there was a modest move towards more organically grown foods. Daily exercise had always formed part of his routine.

Twelve weeks following his MRI confirmation of pancreatic cancer and eight weeks following the onset of Salvestrol supplementation an ultrasound indicated slight shrinkage of the pancreatic tumour. A follow up MRI confirmed the shrinkage and revealed concurrent shrinkage of the kidney tumour. Again no biopsies were taken. Salvestrol supplementation was maintained along with his usual daily supplements. No further changes were made to diet or lifestyle.

Three months following his diagnosis of pancreatic cancer and in light of the results from his last medical imaging his mood improved quite dramatically. He was no longer overcome by the fear of his prognosis.

Four months later and six months after starting Salvestrol supplementation a further ultrasound found no evidence of pancreatic or kidney cancer. Given this surprising result an MRI was scheduled. The MRI confirmed the finding. Due to this highly unusual finding a second MRI was performed which also confirmed the finding – no evidence of pancreatic or kidney cancer was found. An astonished oncologist told him that he was cancer free and that the kidney had healed very well. A follow up flexible cystoscopy, ultrasound and MRI were scheduled in a year's time.

FOLLOW UP:

Current health status:	enjoying good health – cancer free
Time since diagnosis:	32 months
Months in remission:	16

After being declared cancer free he decreased his daily Salvestrol supplementation to one 2,000 point capsule per day. He has commenced a daily, one hour walk and modified his diet to include organically grown foods whenever practical to do so. He is feeling great and enjoying good health. Twelve months following his cancer free status, he reported that he feels ten years younger and his recurrent problems with nail fungus (onychomycosis with concurrent paronychia) have also been resolved. Salvestrol cream was applied for this purpose.

As the date of his one year follow up flexible cystoscopy, ultrasound and MRI approached Salvestrol supplementation was increased to two capsules comprising a total daily intake of 4,000 Salvestrol points and then three capsules for a daily intake of 6,000 Salvestrol points. The one year flexible cystoscopy found no evidence of bladder cancer. Ultrasound found no evidence of pancreatic cancer or kidney cancer. His cancer free status was confirmed and it was felt that there was no need for an MRI. He will be tested again in a year's time.

At the time of his diagnosis he was given a life expectancy of 10 to 20 weeks. He has now exceeded that by between 12 to 22 months through nothing other than addressing a dietary deficiency.

RECURRENT, NON-MUSCLE INVASIVE BLADDER CANCER[8]

Date of initial diagnosis:	June, 2000
Age at initial diagnosis:	55
Sex:	male
Country of residence:	England
Salvestrol points per day:	4,000 points
Time from start of Salvestrol use to being told he was cancer free:	5 months

Time in remission with
no evidence of cancer: 19 months

A 55-year-old male noticed blood in his urine. He visited his doctor and a cystoscopic examination of his bladder was arranged. This examination revealed hundreds of small, papillary tumours (small tumours that are shaped like a nipple or the head of a mushroom). He was diagnosed with non muscle invasive (superficial) bladder cancer. Surgery was recommended to remove the tumours and he accepted this recommendation. Following surgery, cystoscopic examinations with further surgery if necessary were scheduled at six month intervals to monitor and control disease progression. No other form of treatment was prescribed.

Cystoscopic examinations were conducted every six months. However, surgical removal of the recurrent tumours was scheduled every twelve months. Recurrent tumours continued to be visible through cystoscopic examination for a period of six years and were surgically removed annually. One month following his sixth surgery he learned about Salvestrols from a friend. He began supplementing his diet with 4,000 Salvestrol points per day divided between the three daily meals. Salvestrol supplementation was the only change made to his daily routine. There was no dietary change, no change in exercise or lifestyle, no further supplements were taken and no prescription treatments were used.

Five months after starting to supplement his diet with Salvestrols a cystoscopic examination was scheduled. Cystoscopy revealed no tumours or cancerous tissue. This was the first clean cystoscopic examination since his diagnosis over six years ago. His doctor informed him that he was in remission. The Salvestrols had been given to him by a friend and shortly after receiving this good news he stopped supplementing with Salvestrols as he felt that they were no longer necessary.

He continued to be monitored using cystoscopy. This was initially done at six months and then on an annual basis. Nineteen months after being declared cancer free he was referred for bladder cystoscopy. The result was positive and a follow up MRI was scheduled and showed evidence of a recurrence of his bladder cancer. The cancer was now located in the right ureter (the tube leading from the kidney to the bladder). He was advised that surgery would be necessary and both the ureter and kidney would need to be removed. A week later, surgery was done and his affected ureter and kidney were removed. Immediately after his recovery from surgery he started to supplement his diet with Salvestrols (3,000 points per day). This level of supplementation was maintained for eight months and then reduced to 2,000 points per day for another four months at which point Salvestrol supplementation was stopped. There were no changes to diet or lifestyle during this time.

FOLLOW UP:

Current health status: *prostate cancer risk being monitored*

Time since diagnosis:	*152 months*
Months in remission from being told he was free of his bladder cancer to diagnosis of his kidney cancer:	*19*
Months in remission from being told he was free of his kidney cancer:	*52*

He has continued to be monitored on an annual basis. After his kidney surgery he has remained in remission for over four years. Fifty-two months after his surgery cystoscopy has not found any recurrence of bladder cancer but a routine prostate specific antigen (PSA) test indicated an elevated level (8.2 ng/ml). He was told that he would be re-tested in four weeks and if the PSA level remained elevated he will be scheduled for a biopsy. He has started Salvestrol supplementation again at a level of 6,000 points per day. At the time of writing his second PSA test result indicated a level of 5 ng/ml which is marginally outside of normal limits for his age. No biopsy is scheduled and no treatment is being considered. His PSA level will continue to be monitored. If he does have prostate cancer these early results indicate that it is being controlled by the Salvestrols.

This man appears to have responded exceptionally well to Salvestrols. It is a shame that he has not been consistent in his supplementation. He initially stopped taking Salvestrols after being told he was free of cancer because he did not feel that they were necessary any more. However, given the state of the art in cancer detection, it can be very difficult to determine the full extent of one's cancer. Remission may mean that an unseen tumour(s) is just below the level of detection. Given this, it is important to continue taking a maintenance level of Salvestrols after achieving remission to ensure that any undetected areas of cancer are controlled. Also it is important to engage in dietary change comprising abundant, organic fruits and vegetables and some daily exercise in addition to Salvestrol supplementation.

CHAPTER NOTES:

1. *Cancer: New Registrations and Deaths 2000: Revised Edition*. New Zealand Health Information Service, Ministry of Health, Wellington, 2004.
2. Cancer Research UK. Bladder cancer incidence statistics. http://www.cancerresearchuk.org/cancer-info/cancerstats/types/bladder/incidence/uk-bladder-cancer-incidence-statistics
3. Pan CC, Chang YH, Chen KK, Yu HJ, Sun CH, Ho DM: Prognostic significance of the 2004 WHO/ISUP classification for prediction of recurrence, progression, and cancer-specific mortality of non-muscle-invasive urothelial tumors of the urinary bladder: a clinicopathologic study of 1,515 cases. *Am J Clin Pathol*. 2010; 133(5): 788-95.
4. Herr HW, Donat SM, Reuter VE: Management of low grade papillary bladder tumors. *J Urol*. 2007; 178(4 Pt 1):1201-5.

5. Cancer Research UK. Bladder cancer statistics and outlook. http://cancerhelp.cancerresearchuk.org/type/bladder-cancer/treatment/bladder-cancer-statistics-and-outlook#general
6. Schaefer, B. A. (2013). Case Study: Low grade papillary urothelial carcinoma, kidney cancer and pancreatic cancer. *International Journal of Phytotherapy,* **1**:2, 13.
7. Artinyan A, Soriano PA, Prendergast C et al. The anatomic location of pancreatic cancer is a prognostic factor for survival. *HPB (Oxford)* 2008; 10: 371–376.
8. Schaefer BA, Hoon LT, Burke DM, et al: Nutrition and Cancer: Salvestrol case studies. *J Orthomol Med*, 2007; 22: 177-182.

3.
BREAST CANCER

Breast cancer, as one might imagine, is a cancer that starts in the tissues of the breast. In Canada and the UK breast cancer is the most frequently occurring cancer in women. In Canada the 2007 cancer statistics indicate that there were a total of 21,006 new cases of breast cancer diagnosed and this represents 13% of all cancer diagnoses and 27% of all cancer diagnoses for women (breast cancer incidence for men was extremely uncommon by comparison)[1]. In the UK the 2009 cancer statistics indicate that there were a total of 48,788 new cases of breast cancer diagnosed and this represents 15% of all cancer diagnoses and 31% of all cancer diagnoses for women (like Canada the incidence of breast cancer in UK men is rare by comparison)[2,3].

Breast cancer typically starts in the glandular tissues of the breast (adenocarcinoma), but cancer originating in the ducts (ductal carcinoma) or lobules (lobular carcinoma) are also common. With the very high incidence of breast cancer, it is fortunate that breast cancer does not represent an immediate threat to life. It is the breast cancer metastases to life sustaining organs such as the liver, lung or brain that is the primary concern of anyone diagnosed with this disease. Given this, it is hard to comprehend why a search for metastases is so seldomly conducted prior to embarking on a treatment plan for the breast cancer. Nevertheless, the five-year survival figures for breast cancer are quite good by comparison to the cancers that directly affect life sustaining organs. In the UK, across all breast cancers, those that have been diagnosed have an 85% chance of being alive at the end of five years compared with those that have not had a cancer diagnosis.[4] Canada reports that women who have been diagnosed with breast cancer have an 88% chance of being alive at the end of five years compared with those that have not had cancer.[5]

BREAST CANCER, STAGE 1[6]

Date of diagnosis:	August, 2007
Age at diagnosis:	76
Sex:	female
Country of residence:	Canada
Salvestrol points per day:	1400 points
Time from start of Salvestrol use to being told she was cancer free:	1 month
Time in remission with no evidence of cancer:	60 months

BREAST CANCER

At the age of 76, a woman discovered six lumps at the surface of her right breast while showering. She saw her family physician and was referred to a dermatologist. The dermatologist ordered a biopsy which came back negative for cancer. Her family physician requested a second biopsy which came back positive for breast cancer. A diagnosis of stage 1 breast cancer was made although with 6 cancerous lumps a diagnosis of stage 2 breast cancer would have been more common. She was not informed about the specific type of breast cancer. Treatment using the pharmaceutical aromatase inhibitor, Femara® (letrozole), 2.5 mg daily was recommended, but the woman declined this treatment.

Upon hearing of her diagnosis a friend suggested that she supplement her diet with Salvestrols. She decided to try Salvestrol supplementation for three weeks. She took a daily intake of 1,400 Salvestrol points consisting of 700 Salvestrol points with her breakfast and 700 Salvestrol points before bed. She experienced no side effects and took no additional supplements, alternative treatments, or prescription medications. She maintained her existing diet and lifestyle – she had always had a well-balanced diet and had always included daily walks as part of her routine.

Through breast self-examination she discovered that after 10-12 days of Salvestrol supplementation the lumps had started to shrink. During the third week of Salvestrol supplementation she could not feel any lumps in her breast. She did not experience any breast pain.

One month after her breast cancer diagnosis her family physician ordered both computerised tomography (CT) and mammogram X-ray scans. No cancer was found on either scan. Once again Femara® (2.5 mg once per day) was prescribed, this time to protect against recurrence of the cancer. She stopped Salvestrol supplementation and took the Femara® for a period of two years. During this time she was monitored every three months. Throughout the two year period of taking Femara® she suffered from nausea and dizziness. Her doctor informed her that these were side effects of Femara® and upon hearing this she stopped taking it. At this point she again started taking Salvestrols but at an intake of 1,000 or 2,000 Salvestrol points per day.

The lack of side effects with Salvestrol supplementation was a deciding factor in her decision to decline further Femara® and resume Salvestrol supplementation. She says that with Salvestrol supplementation "it's like you don't know you are even taking anything and it still is doing its job." She was happy with her decision and pleased to be free of side effects.

FOLLOW UP:

Current health status:	recurrent breast cancer five years after the original diagnosis while off Salvestrols
Time since diagnosis:	65 months
Months in remission:	60 months

After a remarkably quick response to Salvestrol supplementation and a rapid return to good health (one month from diagnosis of breast cancer to being declared cancer free) she commenced a two year prescription of Femara® followed by a 4.5 month period of Salvestrol supplementation that varied between 1,000 and 2,000 points per day. At this point she stopped taking Salvestrols. From this point forward she took no prescription drugs or Salvestrols to guard against breast cancer recurrence and no other nutritional supplements.

After being cancer-free for 5 years she was once again diagnosed with breast cancer. She is currently pursuing conventional treatment for breast cancer. It is unfortunate that she stopped taking Salvestrols as a preventative and even more unfortunate that she has not commenced a therapeutic intake of Salvestrols now that she has recurrent breast cancer. Given her incredibly rapid response to Salvestrol supplementation during her first diagnosis, it would seem a reasonable assumption that she would again respond favourably.

BREAST CANCER, STAGE 3[7]

Date of diagnosis:	*January, 2007*
Age at diagnosis:	*50*
Sex:	*female*
Country of residence:	*Canada*
Salvestrol points per day:	*3500 points for 3 months, then 2100 points for 5 months (average daily intake over 8 months 2,625)*

*Time from start of Salvestrol use to being
told she was cancer free:*   8 months
*Time in remission with
no evidence of cancer:*   65 months

A 50-year-old woman was experiencing pain in her upper chest and tiredness. She visited her doctor and a lump was detected in her left breast. She was referred for ultrasound imaging. The imaging revealed a 2.5 cm tumour in her left breast and a subsequent biopsy confirmed a diagnosis of breast cancer. She was told, following a more comprehensive evaluation that she was classified as stage 3 breast cancer, but she was not informed of the specific type of breast cancer. Concurrent with the breast cancer diagnosis, she suffered from hypothyroidism.

Her oncologist recommended chemotherapy, surgical removal of the tumour (lumpectomy) and radiotherapy. She decided against the chemotherapy but agreed to the surgery and radiotherapy. A surgery date was scheduled for exactly one month after the diagnosis had been confirmed. She was given a prescription for Tylenol® 3 (2 tablets at onset of pain) to manage the pain and discomfort.

After her initial visit to her doctor she mentioned her situation to a friend who recommended that she supplement her diet with Salvestrols. She began to take Salvestrols the day before receiving her diagnosis. She took a total of 3,500 Salvestrol points per day divided between the three daily meals. This level of Salvestrol supplementation was carried out for three months.

After reading about the discovery of Salvestrols and the research behind the discovery she embarked on an organic, vegan diet (vegetables, greens, fruits, juices, wheatgrass and tea) and an exercise program of walking and yoga. She also took Salvestrol co-factors: biotin, 300mcg; niacin, amount unknown; magnesium by way of a calcium/magnesium tablet, amount unknown; iron, 1oz., amount unknown; and Vitamin C, 1,000 mg. To this her naturopathic physician added selenium (200mcg) to her daily supplementation.

While waiting for her surgery date she noticed through breast self-examination that the tumour was softening, the texture was changing and the tumour was progressively decreasing in size. In spite of the rapid changes noticed in the breast cancer while she was taking Salvestrols, her surgeon carried out a surgical lumpectomy. At surgery a tumour was removed. It measured 2 x 1.3 x 0.7 cm. This tumour was approximately half the diameter of the tumour that was originally seen during the initial ultrasound imaging. The post-surgical pathology report indicated that the lymph nodes under her arm that were removed during surgery were free of cancer. A hematology panel showed all results to be within normal limits.

One month following the surgery radiotherapy commenced. Radiotherapy was administered once each workday for 30 days as a precaution against recurrence. Radiation therapy to the breast for early stage breast cancer is part of the standard of care for breast cancer in the UK, New Zealand, the United States and Canada, as well as many other countries. The reason it is given is that studies clearly show that the combination of a breast cancer lumpectomy followed by radiation results in a reduced local recurrence rate (to the same breast) as compared to just performing a lumpectomy. However, there is no evidence that it reduces the likelihood of occurrence of either regional metastases or distant metastases and there is no evidence that it increases the likelihood of survival. Furthermore, long-term adverse effects are not uncommon.

Three months following the onset of Salvestrol supplementation she reduced the daily intake to 2,100 points per day. Again these Salvestrol points were divided between the three daily meals. This level of supplementation was maintained for the next five months.

Eight months after surgery she was deemed cancer free. She experienced no pain and little tiredness. Thirteen months after surgery she reported that she remained cancer free with no pain and little tiredness. She still suffered from hypothyroidism. The tumour shrinkage that she experienced during the one month wait for surgery seems attributable to her Salvestrol supplementation, as well as her focus on nutrition and exercise.

FOLLOW UP:

Current health status:	*enjoying good health – cancer free*
Time since diagnosis:	*72 months*
Months in remission:	*65 months*

She has now had 5 years of remission and is feeling great and enjoying excellent health. She has maintained her dietary change, takes an hour of exercise each day and continues with her yoga practice throughout her remission to prevent recurrence.

BREAST CANCER, AGGRESSIVE STAGE 3[8]

Date of diagnosis: May, 2006
Age at diagnosis: 36
Sex: female
Country of residence: England
Salvestrol points per day: 1,000 points for 1 month, 2,000 points for 1.5 months, then 2,350 points (average daily intake over 5 months 1,975)
Time from start of Salvestrol use to cancer undetectable: 5 months
Time in remission with no evidence of cancer: 27 months

An active 36-year-old woman visited her physician after noticing that pain in her right side was interfering with her ability to carry on with her fitness class. There were two palpable lumps, one in her breast and one in a lymph node. She was referred to an oncologist and magnetic resonance imaging (MRI), a mammogram X-ray scan, blood tests and biopsies of the two lumps were arranged. The results of the biopsies combined with the imaging data and blood test results converged on a diagnosis of aggressive, stage 3 breast cancer. A 3-5 cm tumour had been found under the right breast and a larger tumour was found in an underarm lymph node. The breast tumour 'looked the size of a golf ball on the image'.

Her oncologist informed her that her situation was 'really, really serious' and an aggressive treatment plan was necessary. The plan consisted of eight sessions of chemotherapy (four of intravenous Doxil® (doxorubicin), one every three weeks, plus four of intravenous Taxotere® (docetaxel) one every three weeks) followed by surgical removal of the tumours, radiotherapy and then long term use of Tamoxifen®. This is a standard treatment plan, however, it does point out the shortcomings of each component, the chemotherapy, the surgery and the radiation as none of them are deemed sufficiently effective in isolation to merit avoiding the other additional treatments.

She received this treatment plan with trepidation but through befriending a woman that was diagnosed the same day with a less aggressive, stage 2 breast cancer, she found the courage to accept the plan and commence treatment. The first of the chemotherapy sessions commenced soon after.

The first chemotherapy session left her feeling very poorly. Before her second chemotherapy session someone told her about Salvestrols. Although sceptical about how these capsules could possibly help with her situation she began to supplement her diet with Salvestrols taking a daily intake of 1,000

Salvestrol points. She was very surprised when the pain associated with the tumours subsided and shortly thereafter the tumours began shrinking quickly. This was an enormous boost to her morale and she began to feel that 'she was going to be OK.' She began to find out more about Salvestrols and after reading as much as she could she switched to an organic diet and began using organic deodorant, shampoo, soap, cleaners, etc. She also began to minimise her exposure to possible CYP1B1 inhibitors. She increased her daily intake of Salvestrols to 2,000 points per day and made sure that she was obtaining Salvestrol cofactors through diet and supplementation. Enthused about how much better she was feeling she told her new 'chemo friend', as she referred to her, about Salvestrols but her friend insisted that the oncologist knew what was best for her.

She returned for her third chemotherapy session and was examined by her oncologist, as was done prior to each session. The oncologist said that she thought the tumours were gone and referred her for an ultrasound and X-ray mammogram. She was already due to have titanium markers inserted to assist with the surgery that was planned for the end of her chemotherapy sessions. To everyone's surprise the radiologist could find no trace of the tumours through ultrasound and only a shadow was visible on the mammogram. They were consequently unable to place the titanium markers.

Due to the shadow found on the X-ray mammogram she carried on with her chemotherapy sessions.

When she showed up for her fifth chemotherapy session she could not find her new friend. During this session she overheard one of the personnel involved in delivery of the chemotherapy telling a colleague that one in four women die during their chemotherapy sessions. This was enormously distressing to her and in complete contradiction of the published five year survival statistics that report an 85% survival rate. She telephoned her new 'chemo friend' and was informed that she had died. She began to feel very ill after her fifth chemotherapy session, the first course of docetaxel, and also stopped menstruating.

The news of her friend's death, the information that she overheard while receiving her chemotherapy and everyone's surprise that her ultrasound showed no sign of any tumours caused her to lose faith in her physicians. 'If the physicians were not anticipating such an ultrasound result with these drugs why were they administering them?' she wondered. She began to compare her proposed treatment plan to 'Russian Roulette'. She notified her oncologist that she was declining further chemotherapy.

Upon hearing this news the oncology team scheduled another MRI scan and told her that she would have to proceed with radiotherapy and surgery. She was stunned that they wished to proceed with surgery since prior images could not detect tumours. Upon completion of the scan she was informed that she had 'active cancer cells' although no tumours or shadows were visible.

At this point she was very sceptical about her

treatment and she contacted people at two different hospitals to query them as to whether an MRI scan could detect the presence of 'active cancer cells.' She was told that an MRI could not highlight single cells and could only indicate the potential presence of cancer through a visible shadow in the image. She queried her oncology team on this point and they persisted with their recommendation of radiotherapy and surgery although no tumours were present. She declined.

Concerned about the wear and tear on her body from her five chemotherapy sessions she increased her daily intake of Salvestrols to 2,350 points. Four months after declining further conventional treatment she reported that her hair had grown back, she looked good and felt wonderful. She began to menstruate again. She began to actively assist people with cancer in their struggle to regain their health.

FOLLOW UP:

Current health status:	*deceased*
Time since diagnosis:	*n/a*
Months in remission:	*27 months*

Twenty seven months after cancer was not detectable through medical imaging or palpation she died. The cause of her death is not known to us. She did not continue to purchase Salvestrols after the first year of remission.

CHAPTER NOTES:

1. Statistics Canada. Cancer, new cases, by selected primary site of cancer, by sex. http://www.statcan.gc.ca/tables-tableaux/sum-som/l01/cst01/hlth61-eng.htm
2. Cancer Research UK. Cancer Incidence for All Cancers Combined. http://www.cancerresearchuk.org/cancer-info/cancerstats/incidence/all-cancers-combined/
3. Cancer Research UK. Breast Cancer Incidence Statistics. http://www.cancerresearchuk.org/cancer-info/cancerstats/types/breast/incidence/
4. Cancer Research UK. Breast Cancer Survival Statistics. http://www.cancerresearchuk.org/cancer-info/cancerstats/types/breast/survival/
5. Canadian Cancer Society. Breast Cancer Statistics at a Glance. http://www.cancer.ca/Canada-wide/About%20cancer/Cancer%20statistics/Stats%20at%20a%20glance/Breast%20cancer.aspx?sc_lang=en
6. Schaefer, B., Potter G., Wood R., Burke D. Cancer and Related Case Studies Involving Salvestrol and CYP1B1. *J Orthomol Med*, 2012; 27: 131-138.
7. Schaefer BA, Dooner C, Burke DM, Potter GA. Nutrition and Cancer: Further Case Studies Involving Salvestrol. *J Orthomol Med*, 2010; 25, 1: 17-23.
8. Schaefer BA, Hoon LT, Burke DM, Potter GA: Nutrition and Cancer: Salvestrol case studies. *J Orthomol Med*, 2007; 22: 177-182.

4.
COLORECTAL CANCER

Colorectal cancer refers to the various cancers that occur in the colon or rectum. Colorectal cancer has the third highest incidence rate in Canada, with breast cancer for women and prostate cancer for men having the highest incidence and lung cancer having the second highest incidence.[1] According to Statistics Canada, the latest figures are from 2007 and indicate that for males there were 11,211 new cases of colorectal cancer diagnosed in 2007 representing 13% of all new cancer diagnoses for males. For females there were 9,272 new cases of colorectal cancer diagnosed in 2007 representing 12% of all new cancer diagnoses for females.[2] In the United States, colorectal cancer in 2010 is estimated to represent 9% of new cancer diagnoses for men and 9% of new cancer diagnoses for females.[3]

A diagnosis of colorectal cancer will typically mean that you have an adenocarcinoma as this type of cancer accounts for between 90-95% of colorectal diagnoses in Canada.[4] The five year relative survival statistics in Canada are not as favourable as for breast or prostate cancer but are much better than those for lung cancer. Those men that have been diagnosed have a 63% chance of being alive at the end of five years compared with those that have not had a cancer diagnosis while those women that have been diagnosed have a 64% chance of being alive at the end of five years compared with those that have not had a cancer diagnosis.[1] The figures for the United States, for men and women combined, are comparable with a 64% chance of being alive at the end of five years compared with those that have not had a cancer diagnosis.[3]

POSSIBLE COLON CANCER[5] – NO BIOPSY DONE

Age at diagnosis: 64
Date of diagnosis: February, 2007
Sex: female
Country of residence: Canada
Salvestrol points per day: 3,150 points
Time from start of Salvestrol use to being told she was cancer free: 3 months
Time in remission with no evidence of cancer: 69 months

After suffering for three years with failing health a 64-year-old woman visited her doctor. Concerned friends had commented that she did not look good. She had been consistently losing weight over this period of time, her abdomen had become progressively more distended, she felt bloated, weak and her skin had taken on a gray/green tone. She was experiencing chronic, sharp pain in her abdomen that was heightened after eating. This pain was sufficiently severe that she was unable to touch her abdomen or lay face down. She had lost 9% of her weight and had a poor appetite, leaving her underweight for her height. She was fatigued to the point of falling asleep by mid-day. She also experienced occasional nausea, vomiting and blood in her stool. A friend that was a registered nurse told her that she suspected colon cancer and encouraged her to visit her doctor. Her doctor, after conducting a physical exam and review of her symptoms told her that he suspected colon cancer and referred her for testing to confirm his diagnosis.

Her symptom profile was consistent with a diagnosis of colon cancer (blood in her stool, weakness, abdominal pain, bloating, nausea, vomiting, fatigue, weight loss and a skin colouration suggestive of anaemia[5]) but she did not want to pursue conventional treatment for cancer and consequently did not pursue the testing to confirm her diagnosis. It is unfortunate that she did not pursue the testing as a colonoscopy or biopsy could have determined whether the doctor was correct in his diagnosis of colon cancer.

She immediately embarked on an alternative approach to treating her cancer. She began supplementing her diet with 3,150 Salvestrol points per day divided into roughly equal amounts taken with each meal. She maintained this level of Salvestrol supplementation for three months. In addition to Salvestrol supplementation each day she took a multivitamin, one capsule of a fibre and probiotic product 'Colon Green' and one S-adenosyl L-methionine (SAMe) capsule. She also began external application of castor oil packs on the abdomen for four days out of each week.

She responded quickly to the approach that she had put together. After three weeks of Salvestrol supplementation she reported feeling better. Friends and relatives commented that she looked noticeably better by the end of the fifth week. Her abdominal pain and distension subsided by the end of week seven. She began to feel so much better that she returned to her doctor after three months of following this approach to ask for testing to monitor the progression of her colon cancer. After a physical examination the doctor told her that there had been a misdiagnosis and no tests would be ordered.

Seven months after the start of her Salvestrol supplementation her weight had returned to normal and so had her skin colour. She arranged for a privately funded ultrasound investigation to determine whether there were still indications of colon cancer. The ultrasound found no indication of cancer. Upon receipt of this result she reduced her daily Salvestrol intake to 700 points per day. She has great confidence in Salvestrols and attributes her recovery to them.

COLORECTAL CANCER

FOLLOW UP:

Current health status: good health – no evidence of cancer
Time since diagnosis: 72 months
Months in remission: 69

This is a very interesting case in that this woman declined all conventional treatment including the testing necessary to verify whether or not her doctor's suspicion of colon cancer was correct. Clearly her health was severely compromised and the symptom profile would be consistent with that observed in colon cancer. Given the state of her health when she embarked on her nutritional approach she made a remarkable and rapid return to good health. She has now enjoyed more than 5 years with no return of any of her symptoms. She continues to take Salvestrols to prevent a recurrence.

SQUAMOUS CELL CARCINOMA OF THE ANUS

Age at initial diagnosis: 46
Date of initial diagnosis: November, 1997
Sex: male
Country of residence: United States
Salvestrol points per day: 1,000 points
Time from start of Salvestrol use to being told he was cancer free: 3 months
Time in remission with no evidence of cancer: 41 months

At the age of 46, almost 15 years ago, a man was diagnosed with squamous cell carcinoma of the anus. The diagnosis was confirmed with a biopsy and his doctor recommended an abdominoperineal resection (a surgical procedure in which the rectum and anus are removed necessitating a permanent colostomy). He was informed that he may have three years before this procedure would be a necessity. He declined the procedure and embarked upon a series of mental wellness exercises aimed at a positive health outlook along with twice weekly applications of Aldara® (imiquimod) cream which is more commonly prescribed for superficial basal cell carcinomas.

Although he did well using the Aldara® cream the condition persisted and after seven years he was re-diagnosed. This second diagnosis of squamous cell carcinoma of the anus was also confirmed by biopsy. His doctor provided him with the same treatment option and same prognosis as he had for the first diagnosis. Again this man declined the resection and carried on with mental wellness exercises and twice weekly application of Aldara®. Aldara® was minimizing disease progression but proved to be a painful means of accomplishing this objective, as applications would remove the top layers of skin.

After a further three years the disease progressed. Anal lesions were appearing much more frequently and this fellow began to look into options to abdominoperineal resection with colostomy. Sometime later he found a surgeon in New York that had been using a laser surgery for such conditions and went for a consultation.

He was not entirely reassured by the consultation and asked for some time to make a decision.

During his investigation of options to resection this fellow had come across some information about Salvestrols. A friend had passed along a DVD from Health Action Network Society of a lecture by one of the principle scientists behind Salvestrols. By this point a further two years had elapsed since discovering that the anal lesions were appearing more frequently. While trying to decide whether or not to pursue the laser surgery he began supplementing his diet with Salvestrol and began using XM8 cream (i.e., a natural borage oil based cream). He stopped applying Aldara®.

For a three month period he took 1,000 Salvestrol points per day and applied XM8 cream every two to three days. He carried on with his daily mental wellness and physical exercises, took a multi-vitamin, and made dietary changes. He began eating a diet rich in raw vegetables and consumed a "green shake" each day. No pain medications were taken and no additional supplements were consumed.

After a period of six weeks since starting to take the Salvestrols the lesions were no longer visible. At the end of three months his doctor declared him cancer free. Although he requested a biopsy to confirm his cancer free status, his doctor has not obliged. He says, "I thank God that I held onto my belief that there was a better answer and the way I pursued it has really made my life a whole lot more pleasant than the other option [abdominoperineal resection with colostomy] would have posed!"

FOLLOW UP:

Current health status: *good health – cancer free.*
Time since initial diagnosis: *194 months (15 and ¾ years)*
Months in remission: *41*

He has now had 3 years of remission and receives great medical checkups that are free of concerns. He has maintained his Salvestrol supplementation and has replaced the XM8 cream with Salvestrol cream. He continues with his daily, physical and mental wellness exercises, maintains a healthy diet and an optimistic attitude towards health.

CHAPTER NOTES:

1. Canadian Cancer Society. Colorectal Cancer Statistics at a Glance. http://www.cancer.ca/Canada-wide/About%20 cancer/Cancer%20statistics/Stats%20at%20a%20 glance/Colorectal%20cancer.aspx?sc_lang=en
2. Statistics Canada. Cancer, new cases, by selected primary site of cancer, by sex. http://www.statcan.gc.ca/tables-tableaux/sum-som/l01/cst01/hlth61-eng.htm
3. American Cancer Society. Cancer Facts and Figures 2012. http://www.cancer.org/acs/groups/content/@epidemiologysurveilance/documents/document/acspc-031941.pdf
4. Canadian Cancer Society. Canadian Cancer Encyclopedia, Colorectal cancer overview. http://info.cancer.ca/cce-ecc/default.aspx?cceid=627&Lang=E&toc=13#Diagnosis

5. Schaefer BA, Dooner C, Burke DM, Potter GA. Nutrition and Cancer: Further Case Studies Involving Salvestrol. *J Orthomol Med,* 2010; 25, 1: 17-23.
6. Canadian Cancer Society. Canadian Cancer Encyclopedia, Signs and symptoms of colorectal cancer. http://info.cancer.ca/cce-ecc/default.aspx?lf=colorectal&cceid=609&rk=64914833&fp=file%253a%252f%252fcispublicweb%252fe_html%252f13_4004.html&sqg=2aa29f4d-f9ef-4dc7-b3ff-e4a60aa06365&toc=13
7. Schaefer, B., Potter G., Wood R., Burke D. Cancer and Related Case Studies Involving Salvestrol and CYP1B1. *J Orthomol Med,* 2012; 27: 131-138.

5
CHRONIC LYMPHOCYTIC LEUKAEMIA

Leukaemia is a cancer of the blood forming system found in the bone marrow, characterized by an abnormal increase of immature white blood cells in the bloodstream. Leukaemia is a broad term covering a spectrum of diseases. In turn, it is part of the even broader group of diseases affecting the blood, bone marrow, and lymphoid system, which are all known as hematological neoplasms. In the next chapter, we will look at a case of Hodgkin's disease, which involves cells in the lymph system, but does not result in an increase of these cells in the bloodstream, as do the leukaemias. In addition to an elevation of certain abnormal white blood cells in the bloodstream, leukaemias may also show up as lumps or bumps in lymph nodes throughout the body as seen in the case to be discussed.

There are many different types of leukemia, which are classified by which type of cell is involved and whether or not the disease is considered acute or chronic. For example, there are acute and chronic lymphocytic leukemias and acute and chronic myelogenous leukemias. The normal course of these untreated diseases are quite different with the expected survival times also being quite different. The most benign type of leukemia is chronic lymphocytic leukemia, which we will discuss in this chapter. These patients often can live for years with their disease, which is characterized by an increase in a certain type of abnormal lymphocytes in the bloodstream.

Leukaemia (all of the various types of leukaemia combined) is among the top 10 most commonly diagnosed cancers in the UK for both males and females. According to Cancer Research UK, the latest statistics are from 2009 and indicate that for males there were 4844 new cases of leukaemia diagnosed in 2009 representing 3% of all new cancer diagnoses for males, while for females, there were 3458 new cases of leukaemia diagnosed in 2009 representing 2.2% of all new cancer diagnoses for females.[1]

Chronic lymphocytic leukaemia (CLL) is the most common form of leukaemia representing about 35% of leukaemia diagnoses. It is more often diagnosed in older people with 75% of diagnoses in people over the age of 60. In CLL it is the lymphocytes that are cancerous. CLL is not often cured but since CLL develops slowly in many people it can often be controlled.[2] Consistent with the poor cure rate, CLL has a variable prognosis and an exceptionally rare rate of spontaneous remission, especially with those that were not diagnosed in the early stage of disease progression.[3] In England, for those diagnosed with chronic lymphocytic leukaemia, the men had a 44% chance of being alive at the end of five years compared with those that have not had a cancer diagnosis, while the five year relative survival rate for females was 52%.[4]

CHRONIC LYMPHOCYTIC LEUKAEMIA[6]

Age at diagnosis:	80
Date of diagnosis:	October, 2010
Sex:	female
Country of residence:	England
Salvestrol points per day:	2,000 points
Time from start of Salvestrol use to being told she was cancer free:	3 months
Time in remission with no evidence of cancer:	22 months
Rate of spontaneous remission with CLL:	1%

In April of 2012 my friend and colleague, Gerry Potter, introduced me to an 81 year-old woman in England that had suffered from Chronic Lymphocytic Leukaemia. At the age of 80 she had developed an 'egg sized' tumour on the left side of her neck. She went to her doctor, blood tests were ordered and a referral was made to an oncologist and an ear, nose and throat specialist. One month following her initial visit to the doctor she was seen by an ear, nose and throat specialist who took a biopsy of the tumour. During the following three weeks her condition deteriorated. She was having discomfort and difficulties sleeping due to the swelling and tenderness of the lymph glands in her groin and armpits. A scan of her neck and abdomen was arranged revealing swelling in all lymph glands. Blood was sent to the lab for analysis.

Two months later, based on the biopsy, the blood work, and the scan, a diagnosis of chronic lymphocytic leukaemia was made. With swelling in all lymph glands and tumour development, this was an advanced stage of chronic lymphocytic leukaemia. She was told that she probably had this condition for many years prior to her diagnosis. As for a prognosis she was told that it was very difficult to provide her with an accurate prognosis, she may live for two days, two weeks, two months or two years. Treatment options were discussed and declined.

For two months following her diagnosis her condition continued to decline. Severe pain developed in her throat causing great difficulty with swallowing and sleeping. Consequently she ate very little and began to lose weight. Her ear, nose and throat specialist took a biopsy of the ulcer that had developed on her tonsil and this biopsy confirmed that it was part of the chronic lymphocytic leukaemia. Her oncologist referred her for radiotherapy.

While waiting for the results of the tonsil biopsy her condition continued to decline. She noticed that a tumour was beginning to show on the right side of her neck and the swelling in the groin and armpits continued. During this time she met with an old friend and began telling her about her situation. As it turned out this friend of hers was also a close friend of Gerry Potter's mother so she was well versed in the Salvestrol research. Gerry's mother was contacted and Salvestrols were made available.

By the time she heard about Salvestrols six months had elapsed since her first visit to the doctor for this condition. She began taking two thousand Salvestrol points per day. She increased her consumption of fruit and vegetables and decided to reduce stress in her life by dropping some of her obligations.

After her first month of Salvestrol supplementation she was feeling much better. The tumours in her neck had started to soften and shrink and the swelling had subsided to the point that she was getting far more sleep. This quick progress coincided with her appointment for radiotherapy. She attended the appointment and told the radiotherapist that she was feeling so much better that she would rather forego the radiotherapy and see if she continued to improve without it. The radiotherapist respected her wishes and said that she could always come back for radiotherapy if she felt that she needed it.

She was pleased that she was able to avoid the radiotherapy and after two months of continued Salvestrol supplementation, the tumours in her neck had almost disappeared. At the end of three months of Salvestrol supplementation the tumours were completely gone, the pain in her throat from the ulcer was gone, and the swelling in her groin and armpits was gone. She returned to her oncologist for further testing and was informed that there was no evidence of cancer – she was all clear. Her oncologist expressed great surprise at her current good health and weight gain.

Upon hearing this news she carried on with her more relaxed lifestyle and her dietary focus on increased fruit and vegetable consumption but stopped taking Salvestrols. After a period of a few months she returned to Salvestrol supplementation and started taking 1,000 Salvestrol points per day. She is feeling great and hopes that her experience will be of benefit to others.

FOLLOW UP:

Current health status:	*enjoying good health – cancer free*
Time since diagnosis:	*28 months*
Months in remission:	*22*

She has had a remarkable recovery from her illness – remarkable not only in the speed of her recovery but also in the low dose of Salvestrols that she was taking. She has now had 22 months of remission and is feeling great. She maintains her dietary change and Salvestrol supplementation. With continued Salvestrol supplementation she should be able to avoid recurrence.

CHAPTER NOTES:

1. Cancer Research UK. Cancer Incidence for Common Cancers. http://info.cancerresearchuk.org/cancerstats/incidence/commoncancers/
2. Cancer Research UK. Cancer Incidence for Common Cancers. Statistics and outlook for chronic lymphocytic leukaemia (CLL). http://cancerhelp.cancerresearchuk.org/type/cll/treatment/statistics-and-outlook-for-chronic-lymphocytic-leukaemia
3. Del Giudice I, Chiaretti S, Tavolaro S, De Propris MS, Maggio R, Mancini F, et al. Spontaneous regression of chronic lymphocytic leukemia: clinical and biologic features of 9 cases. *Blood*, 2009, 114(3):638–46.
4. Cancer Research UK. Statistics and outlook for chronic lymphocytic leukaemia (CLL). http://cancerhelp.cancerresearchuk.org/type/cll/treatment/statistics-and-outlook-for-chronic-lymphocytic-leukaemia
5. Schaefer, B., Potter G., Wood R., Burke D. Cancer and Related Case Studies Involving Salvestrol and CYP1B1. *J Orthomol Med*, 2012; 27: 131-138.

6.
HODGKIN LYMPHOMA
(ALSO KNOWN AS HODGKIN'S DISEASE)

The body makes several types of blood cells. Red blood cells mainly help to carry oxygen to all cells of the body. The white blood cells are primarily involved with the immune system in the body, which helps to defend against an invading microorganism. The white cells are divided into several groups, including lymphocytes, which are further divided into T cells and B cells.

Hodgkin's lymphoma (HL) starts in the lymphatic system. HL almost always starts in the B cells. In Canada, the incidence of Hodgkin's lymphoma is much lower than the incidence of non-Hodgkin lymphoma. Statistics Canada estimates that for Canadian males there will be 510 new cases of Hodgkin lymphoma in 2012 representing 0.52% of all new cancer diagnoses for males while for females there will be 430 new cases representing 0.48% of all new cancer diagnoses for Canadian females.[1]

Hodgkin's disease is classified into 4 stages with the 1st stage showing the least disease and the 4th stage showing the most disease. Stage I involves the presence of cancer in one group of lymph nodes either above or below the diaphragm. Stage II involves two or more groups of lymph nodes either above or below the diaphragm. Stage III involves two or more lymph nodes both above and below the diaphragm and stage IV involves organs beyond the lymph nodes, such as the liver or lung. These stages relate to prognosis with the prognosis getting worse as the stage increased. Hodgkin's lymphoma is further classified as A or B with A characterized by no systemic symptoms and B characterized by systemic symptoms, such as fever, weight loss or night sweats. The cancer journey discussed below was 3B, which generally has a poor prognosis.

The incidence of HL is highest in older adults, that is, those over the age of 55 and in younger adults between the mid-teens to the mid-30s. The prognosis for patients is variable based on the stage of the disease and the presence of various prognostic factors such as having stage 4 disease, being over 45 years old, being male, and specific levels of albumin, hemoglobin, white blood cells and lymphocytes. People diagnosed in Canada with HL have an 85% chance of being alive in five years relative to people that have not received a cancer diagnosis. However, the relative five year survival rate is variable across the various stages of HL with a relative five year survival rate of greater than 90% for stage 0 and a relative five year survival rate of around 65% for stage 4.[2]

HODGKIN LYMPHOMA, STAGE 3B[3]

Age at diagnosis: 66
Date of diagnosis: April, 2007
Sex: male
Country of residence: Canada
Salvestrol points per day: 4,000 points
Time from start of Salvestrol use to being told he was cancer free: 1 ¼ months
Time in remission with no evidence of cancer: 52 months

A 66 year old man underwent quadruple by-pass surgery. The surgeon noticed abnormalities in chest lymph nodes during the surgical procedure and referred him to a cancer specialist for follow-up. Tumours were found in the lymph nodes of the neck, chest, abdomen and groin with some approaching 3 cm in diameter. At the time of the examination, the patient had suffered significant loss of appetite with consequent weight loss, as well as pain in the area of his neck, stomach, and groin. The pain was significant enough to require 16 to 20 Tylenol® 3 tablets per day to control the pain. A biopsy was obtained as part of an endoscopic examination and resulted in a diagnosis of stage 3B Hodgkin Lymphoma. He was advised by his physicians that his cancer was sufficiently advanced that he had only one to two years before the disease would end his life.

Subsequent to his diagnosis a referral for chemotherapy was given. Chemotherapy was administered and maintained for a period of six months. In British Columbia, Canada, where this fellow was treated, ABVD is the standard chemotherapy[4]. ABVD is a mixture of chemotherapies containing: A- doxorubicin (Adriamycin®); B- bleomycin (Blenoxane®); V- vinblastine (Velban®); and D- dacarbazine (DTIC-Dome®). No radiation therapy was given.

The chemotherapy proved to be very difficult for him to tolerate, however, he completed the full course. After six months of chemotherapy a positron emission tomography (PET) scan revealed a lesion on his pancreas. This proved to be benign. In addition, the scan revealed that the tumours in his neck, abdomen and groin remained and those in the neck and abdomen showed signs of continued growth during the chemotherapy. No further treatment was provided.

A healthcare practitioner that was assisting this man with some of his symptoms suggested that he try Salvestrols. One month following his chemotherapy he began taking Salvestrol (1,000 point) capsules. Two capsules were taken in the morning and two were taken in the evening for a total daily intake of 4,000 Salvestrol points. This was maintained for 38 days which is the number of days that two bottles of 75 capsules each would last at this level of intake (this man was concurrently suffering from financial hardship and accepted a gift of two bottles but was reluctant to accept further charity). There was no concurrent treatment, no dietary changes were made and no additional supplements were used. His appetite returned to normal quite quickly after starting to take Salvestrols and he began to regain the weight that he had lost.

When he had finished the two bottles of Salvestrols, 38 days after starting, he was due to visit his oncologist. His oncologist informed him that the tumours that remained after the chemotherapy was completed were now gone and that he was in remission. He has been followed up by his oncologist every three months. Friends stepped in to supply him with further Salvestrols, which he initially accepted but then declined. He was unable to purchase them for himself due to the financial constraints resulting from his illness. He attributes his remission to his use of Salvestrols and intends to continue taking Salvestrols as soon as his financial situation improves.

FOLLOW UP:

Current health status: recurrent Hodgkin Lymphoma
Time since diagnosis: 70 months
Months in remission: 52

He has not carried on with Salvestrol supplementation. Whereas his financial situation did improve somewhat he has suffered from some signs of dementia. As he lives alone there is no one to provide him with daily guidance for maintaining his health. His diet and lifestyle remain unchanged from before his original diagnosis. He has been diagnosed with recurrent Hodgkin Lymphoma and is due for further follow up tests at the end of the month. Chemotherapy has been administered and was successful. He is currently due for his 1 year follow up. His medical advisors gave him a one to two year survival estimate upon his initial diagnosis. He has done remarkably better than this as he has remained in remission for over four years and has lived almost six years beyond the date of his initial diagnosis.

CHAPTER NOTES:

1. Statistics Canada. Canadian Cancer Statistics 2012. http://www.cancer.ca/Canada-wide/About%20cancer/~/media/CCS/Canada%20wide/Files%20List/English%20files%20heading/PDF%20-%20Policy%20-%20Canadian%20Cancer%20Statistics%20-%20English/Canadian%20Cancer%20Statistics%202012%20-%20English.ashx
2. Canadian Cancer Society. Canadian Cancer Encyclopedia. Survival Statistics for Hodgkin Lymphoma. http://info.cancer.ca/cce-ecc/default.aspx?Lang=E&toc=19
3. Schaefer BA, Dooner C, Burke DM, Potter GA. Nutrition and Cancer: Further Case Studies Involving Salvestrol. *J Orthomol Med,* 2010; 25, 1: 17-23.
4. BCCA Protocol Summary for Treatment of Hodgkin's Disease with Doxorubicin, Bleomycin, Vinblastine, and Dacarbazine February 1, 2008.

7.
PRIMARY LIVER CANCER

Primary liver cancer is among the top 10 most commonly diagnosed cancers in South Korea for both males and females. Primary liver cancer refers to a cancer which originates in the liver. This is in contrast to secondary or metastatic liver cancers, which originate in another organ or tissue, such as the breast, prostate or lung, and then spread or metastases to the liver.

According to the South Korean National Cancer Center the latest figures are from 2009 and indicate that for males there were 11,913 new cases of liver cancer diagnosed in 2009 representing 12% of all new cancer diagnoses for males. For females there were 4,023 new cases of liver cancer diagnosed in 2009 representing 4.3% of all new cancer diagnoses for females.[1] The outlook for those with liver cancer has not been good. In 2009, for males in South Korea, liver cancer accounted for 19.2% of all cancer deaths while for females, it accounted for 10.9% of all cancer deaths.[2] These mortality percentages for liver cancer are considerably higher than the incidence figures of this disease as shown above.

Primary liver cancer, that is cancer that originates in the liver as opposed to a cancer that has metastasised to the liver, is often associated with viral hepatitis, cirrhosis and/or alcoholism. The prognosis is typically poor. In South Korea the people that were diagnosed with primary liver cancer between 2004 and 2008 had a 23.3% chance of being alive at the end of five years compared with those that have not had a cancer diagnosis.[3]

Primary liver cancer is much more common in South Korea and other countries in South East Asia than it is in North America or Europe. The individual discussed here is from South Korea.

LIVER CANCER – STAGE 2[4]

Age at diagnosis:	73
Date of diagnosis:	October, 2006
Sex:	male
Country of residence:	South Korea
Salvestrol points per day:	4,200 for 4 months, 2,100 for 7 months (average 2864)
Time from start of Salvestrol use to being told he was cancer free:	11 months
Time in remission with no evidence of cancer:	36 months

PRIMARY LIVER CANCER

A 73-year old Korean male who suffered from alcohol-related cirrhosis of the liver began experiencing new symptoms. He lost a lot of weight, experienced nausea, and pain that was at times so severe that he had to crawl to get around in his home. He was spitting up blood (he concurrently suffered from a stomach ulcer and pulmonary tuberculosis) and he noticed an unusual odour associated with his bowel movements.

He was regularly monitored for his cirrhosis and when he attended his next scheduled doctor's appointment with his new symptoms he was referred for a computerised tomography (CT) scan. The CT scan revealed three tumours, one in the centre of the liver in damaged tissue and two in healthy portions of his liver. He was given a diagnosis of stage 2 liver cancers but was not informed of the type of liver cancers. Given the prior diagnosis of alcohol-related cirrhosis there is a high probability that he was suffering from hepatocellular liver cancer as this is the most common form of primary liver cancer and the one most often associated with prior diagnoses of cirrhosis.

The location of the tumours ruled out surgery and due to his age, his concurrent diagnoses and the number of tumours, no chemotherapy or radiotherapy were prescribed. In the absence of standard treatment options he was scheduled for a hepatic artery embolisation one month after being diagnosed as an attempt to downstage the tumours (hepatic artery embolisation is a surgical technique aimed at blocking or restricting blood supply to the tumour).

Around the time of his hepatic artery embolisation,

his son convinced him to begin Salvestrol supplementation. He began taking 4,200 Salvestrol points daily divided between the three daily meals. This level of supplementation was carried out for four months. After four months the daily intake was reduced to 2,100 Salvestrol points divided between the three daily meals. He attempted dietary change but found this particularly difficult and quickly resorted to his typical diet of spicy, salty food.

He did, however, begin a series of lifestyle changes that saw him engaging in daily breathing exercises, chi exercises, stretching exercises, meditation and stress avoidance. In addition, he began receiving intravenous vitamin C injections starting at 30 g per week. This dose was increased through the following weeks, moving in large increments, until reaching 100 g per week. This level was maintained for six months before it was reduced to an ongoing weekly injection of 40 g. Niacin was also added to his wellness plan about four months after his diagnosis. He initially took 250 mg per day for one month and then increased this amount to 500 mg per day for about five months.

Since this man had a variety of concurrent medical problems (stomach ulcer; pulmonary tuberculosis; cirrhosis; and primary liver cancer) he was monitored closely by his healthcare team. He made steady but slow improvement. Eleven months after beginning his Salvestrol supplementation he was declared free of cancer. Even with his other medical problems he reported that he felt very comfortable. Given that hepatic artery embolisation is not a curative procedure, this leaves Salvestrol supplementation, high dose Vitamin C, niacin, exercise and mental outlook as the possible candidates to explain his recovery. He provided the following message to fellow cancer sufferers: "Confidence and belief of being cured is important. People say everything comes from mind. Therefore, I think positive and stable mind is very important. I think we all need confidence that we can overcome any diseases. Anyone can do it!"

FOLLOW UP:

Current health status:	*recurrent liver cancer*
Time since diagnosis:	*76 months*
Months in remission:	*36*

After being declared cancer free he maintained his daily practice of breathing exercises and stretching (yoga) exercises to control his mind and minimise stress. He lost his local supplier of Salvestrols and was unaware of an alternative supply so Salvestrol supplementation ceased. About two years ago he started drinking again and his state of health began to deteriorate quickly. Given the deterioration of his health he was referred for a computerised tomography (CT) scan. The CT scan revealed that his cancer had recurred. Again no treatment was suggested. In the absence of a supply of Salvestrols he has been supplementing his diet with vitamins, doing breathing exercises and yoga. At 80 years of age he now uses a cane and enjoys a good appetite. He is considered stable. By way of his son he has provided the following advice for fellow cancer sufferers: "As we all aware now, cancer is matter of immune system's strength. No matter which part of their body has cancer, he thinks it is more important to strengthen immune system by helping our body's natural healing power. So, our body can heal any disease that one faces. He is sure any disease can be healed. He wants to encourage everyone to face and fight their own disease with confidence, everyone can return to their healthy state."

He has now been resupplied with Salvestrols and we look forward to our next update from him.

CHAPTER NOTES:

1. South Korean National Cancer Center. Cancer Incidence in Korea, 2009. http://ncc.re.kr/english/infor/kccr.jsp
2. South Korean National Cancer Center. Cancer Facts and Figures 2011 in the Republic of Korea. http://ncc.re.kr/english/infor/cff.jsp
3. Jung KW, Park S, Kong HJ, et al: Cancer Statistics in Korea: Incidence, Mortality, Survival and Prevalence in 2008. *Cancer Res Treat*. 2011 March; 43(1): 1–11.
4. Schaefer BA, Dooner C, Burke DM, Potter GA. Nutrition and Cancer: Further Case Studies Involving Salvestrol. *J Orthomol Med*, 2010; 25, 1: 17-23.

8.
PRIMARY LUNG CANCER

Primary lung cancer is a cancer that starts in the lung. Frequently, cancers that begin in other sites, such as the breast, prostate or colon, spread or metastasise to the lungs. These are called secondary cancers. There are two major types of primary lung cancer: non-small cell lung cancer; and small cell lung cancer. Each of these two types is subdivided into three sub-types. Non-small cell lung cancer is the more common type in Canada and in the US. Lung cancer is among the top 10 most commonly diagnosed cancers in Canada for both males and females. According to Statistics Canada the latest figures are from 2007 and indicate that for males there were 12,465 new cases of lung cancer diagnosed in 2007 representing 15% of all new cancer diagnoses for males. For females there were 10,400 new cases of lung cancer diagnosed in 2007 representing 13% of all new cancer diagnoses for females.[1]

While non-small cell lung cancer accounts for about 80% of all lung cancer diagnoses in Canada squamous cell carcinoma of the lung accounts for 30% of the non-small cell lung cancer diagnoses. Squamous cell carcinomas are most common in the bronchial tubes and typically present with coughing up blood (hemoptysis). Although squamous cell carcinomas of the lung have a slightly better prognosis than some other non-small cell carcinomas of the lung, the five year survival rate is only 16%.[2] Lung cancers have a very high rate of mortality. Although lung cancer diagnoses represent 14% of new diagnoses lung cancer deaths represent 27% of all cancer deaths. One is every 13 Canadian men will die of lung cancer while one in every eighteen Canadian women will die of lung cancer.[2]

SQUAMOUS-CELL CARCINOMA OF THE LUNG – STAGE 2-3[3]

Age at diagnosis:	69
Date of diagnosis:	February 2007
Sex:	male
Country of residence:	Canada
Salvestrol points per day:	4200 points
Time from start of Salvestrol use to being told he was cancer free:	6 weeks
Time in remission with no evidence of cancer:	59 months

A 69-year-old male visited his doctor after coughing

up blood. He was not experiencing any pain and felt fine otherwise. His doctor referred him for bronchoscopy. Bronchoscopy detected a seven-centimetre tumour that was adhering to the sternum and chest wall. Enlarged lymph nodes were also detected. The pathology report indicated a diagnosis of stage 2-3 squamous cell carcinoma of the lung. The lung cancer was said to be inoperable. No chemotherapy or radiation treatments were recommended. He was told that his life expectancy was between eight and eighteen months without treatment.

A stepson was well read regarding nutrition and cancer and particularly impressed by the 'China Study' by Colin and Thomas Campbell.[4] This stepson felt that a poor diet and lifestyle had contributed to his stepfather's condition and suggested that he could help his stepfather improve his health through switching his diet to fresh, organic fruit, vegetables and juices that they prepared. Refined sugar, dairy products and meat were eliminated. Concurrent with the dietary change he was encouraged to supplement his diet with Salvestrols. The stepfather, shocked by his diagnosis and prognosis, was motivated to respect his stepson's wishes. A total of 12 of the Salvestrol, 350 point, capsules were taken each day. Four capsules were taken with each meal for a total daily intake of 4,200 Salvestrol points. This level of supplementation was appropriate for his body mass index and was maintained for six weeks.

Benefits were quickly realised. By the end of the first week of dietary change and Salvestrol supplementation he was no longer coughing up blood. Within three weeks his doctor reassessed his statement that the cancer was inoperable and recommended that surgery be booked to remove one lung. At the end of three weeks a biopsy of the largest lymph node was taken following a PET scan and it was found to be negative for cancer. The surgical status of the cancer was changed once again. Although the disease was clearly diminishing at a rapid rate it was now suggested that surgery be booked for the removal of one lobe of the affected lung. One has to wonder why the decision to proceed with surgery was not put on hold given the rapid and dramatic reversal of this disease, but it is fairly common for conventional physicians to rely on conventional treatments, such as surgery, radiation and chemotherapy.

Dietary change and Salvestrol supplementation were maintained and six weeks after commencing this regime surgery was performed. During surgery the tumour was found to be clear of both the sternum and the chest wall and much smaller than anticipated. The lobe was left intact and the shrunken tumour removed along with a couple of suspicious looking lymph nodes.

The postsurgical pathology report indicated that the lymph nodes were not cancerous. The patient was declared free of cancer. Immediately following surgery he reduced the amount of Salvestrol supplementation to six capsules per day (2,100 points), spread across the daily meals and also maintained a diet rich in organic fruit and vegetables.

PRIMARY LUNG CANCER

FOLLOW UP:

Current health status: recurrent squamous cell carcinoma of the lung
Time since diagnosis: 72 months
Months in remission: 59

After being declared cancer free by his attending physician, this fellow finished taking the Salvestrol supplements that he had on hand but did not order more. He maintained his dietary change for a short period of time but gradually moved back to his old eating habits. During this time his stepson moved to another province. This fellow remained in remission for 59 months but then was diagnosed with a recurrence of his squamous cell carcinoma of the lung.

Although he responded exceptionally quickly to dietary changes and the use of Salvestrol supplementation when he was first diagnosed, he did not go back to this protocol when he was once again diagnosed with squamous cell carcinoma of the lung. Instead, he decided to pursue conventional radiation therapy instead. This change of strategy for the recurrent cancer points to the dynamics that surround a very life threatening cancer diagnosis. In the initial cancer diagnosis the stepson was present, concerned and willing to assist. The stepfather, having been told that his life expectancy was now very short, was more than willing to oblige his stepson. Why wouldn't he? The stepson was showing his concern and his suggestions represented no risk whatsoever. With the second diagnosis the stepson was no longer present to express his concern face to face and to present his case for dietary change from this close vantage point. The stepfather clearly engaged in dietary change and Salvestrol supplementation to appease his stepson rather than believing that these changes would benefit his health. It seems clear that he felt that it was the surgery that brought about his original remission so in the absence of his stepsons guidance he chose the conventional approach of radiotherapy. Radiotherapy, in a situation like this is considered palliative by conventional physicians which means that further recurrence will be likely.

It is a shame that no one told him that cancer free means that cancer is not detectable with the technology available for cancer detection. At present, modern technology can only detect the presence of cancer once the cancer has grown to between 10^8 and 10^9 cells (there is an excellent article by Prof. Dan Burke on this point titled "The Silent Growth of Cancer").[5] Had he been aware of this fact he may have been more inclined to carry on with dietary change and Salvestrol supplementation. Given the dramatic response that he experienced when he first commenced dietary change and Salvestrol supplementation, he may well have been able to avoid this recurrence.[6] Nevertheless, after being given a survival estimate of eight to eighteen months by his doctor he remained in remission for 59 months and is still alive 72 months after his original diagnosis.

His stepson has continued to try to persuade him to engage in dietary change and to use Salvestrol supplementation but to no avail.

CHAPTER NOTES:

1. Statistics Canada. Cancer, new cases, by selected primary site of cancer, by sex. http://www.statcan.gc.ca/tables-tableaux/sum-som/l01/cst01/hlth61-eng.htm
2. Canadian Cancer Society. Canadian Cancer Encyclopedia. Lung Cancer Overview. http://info.cancer.ca/cce-ecc/default.aspx?cceid=4240&se=yes&Lang=E
3. Schaefer BA, Hoon LT, Burke DM, et al: Nutrition and Cancer: Salvestrol case studies. *J Orthomol Med*, 2007;22:177-182.
4. Campbell, T. Colin, and Campbell, Thomas M. 2006. *The China Study: The Most Comprehensive Study of Nutrition Ever Conducted and the Startling Implications for Diet, Weight Loss and Long-term Health*. BenBella Books.
5. Burke, MD. (2009). The silent growth of cancer and its implications for nutritional protection. *British Naturopathic Journal*, **26**:1, 15-18.
6. Schaefer, BA. (2012). Case study follow up: lung cancer. *International Journal of Phytotherapy*, **1**:1, 11.

9.
MELANOMA

Malignant melanoma is the most deadly form of skin cancer. In Canada, in 2010, melanoma was one of the top 10 highest incidence cancers for both males and females representing 3% of new cancer diagnoses for each sex.[1] Interestingly melanoma is more likely to occur on the legs of women and on the chest or back of men.[2] Malignant melanomas frequently metastasize and once this occurs, the survival statistics drop dramatically. Once metastases occur, conventional treatment results are very poor.

Early detection of melanoma is very important from a survival perspective. People diagnosed in Canada with melanoma have a 90% chance of being alive in five years relative to people that have not received a cancer diagnosis provided that the diagnosis is made early enough and the cancer is completely removed surgically. However, the relative five year survival rate falls quite dramatically across the various stages of melanoma with a relative five year survival rate of 99% for stage 0 melanoma and a relative five year survival rate of between 10-19% for stage 4 melanoma.[3] Melanomas are staged based on the size and spread of the cancer. A melanoma stage 0 refers to a melanoma in situ (in its original place or position) and is not yet a full malignant melanoma. A stage 4 malignant melanoma is characterized by having spread to distant areas of skin or distant lymph nodes, or to other organs such as the lung, liver or brain. This is called advanced or metastatic melanoma.

MELANOMA – STAGE 4[4]

Age at diagnosis:	94
Date of diagnosis:	May 2006
Sex:	female
Country of residence:	Canada
Salvestrol points per day:	4,000 points per day for 7 months followed by 1,400 points per day for 5 months
Time from start of Salvestrol use to being told she was cancer free:	12 months
Time in remission with no evidence of cancer:	8 months

A 94-year-old woman developed a sore on her foot that was growing and not responding to the treatment supplied by the nurses at her supportive nursing-care facility. Black spots had suddenly appeared on her body and these were also increasing in size. Her doctor was called and a biopsy of the sore was obtained. In consultation with an oncologist a diagnosis of stage 4, metastasised, melanoma was made. Concurrent with this diagnosis she had been suffering from Alzheimer's disease. The treatment that was suggested was hospitalisation, surgery to remove the cancerous sore, a skin graft to close the opening, followed by chemotherapy. Given her age and condition the oncologist did not feel that the skin graft would be successful and this would result in amputation of her foot. Her doctor, oncologist and family concurred that she was unlikely to survive such an intervention. With this decision made the family was told that she would likely live for two weeks and that if she lived longer she would require morphine for pain control. The family asked about what alternative approaches might be followed. The answer was none.

This woman's son had attended a lecture sponsored by Health Action Network Society on Salvestrols and cancer and decided to try them. He also took his mother to the clinic of a Naturopathic College for a consultation. With the assistance of the nursing staff at the care facility she was started on a daily intake of 4,000 Salvestrol points per day divided between the three daily meals. This level of supplementation was maintained for seven months and then reduced to 1,400 Salvestrol points per day for five months. In addition, Salvestrol Cream was applied to the cancerous growth on her foot three times per day. Her diet was changed to an organic, wholesome diet.

The naturopathic physician at the College suggested the following plan: Anti-inflammatory diet (minimal dairy; no tomatoes; no red meat; rice protein in a shake; substitution of berries for sugar and simple carbohydrates; fresh organic fruit juice); Fish Oils 1 g EPA/day; Modified Citrus Pectin 10 g/day; Quercetin 6 capsules/day; Curcumin 4 capsules/day; Vitamin D3 1000 – 1200 Units/day; Reishi 2 g/day; Metagenics-UltraInflamX 2 scoops/day; buffered vitamin C up to 10 g/day or to bowel tolerance; IV vitamin C 2 times/week up to 50 g/session.

At the time that the Salvestrol supplementation and alternative treatment plan commenced she was confined to a wheelchair and unable to put any weight on her foot. She was weak and unable to leave the care facility so the IV vitamin C sessions were abandoned after the initial consultation with the naturopathic physician. Counter to expectation, pain medications were never required. She continued to take medication for her Alzheimer's along with sedatives.

Improvement in her condition was slow and steady. After a few months the melanoma was healing and she was once again able to put some weight on her foot. The black spots that had appeared so suddenly stopped growing and appeared contained. After the passage of a few more months she began walking with the aid of her wheelchair rather than being pushed in her wheelchair. Between six and eight months after starting her Salvestrols supplementation and alternative treatment plan she was symptom free. The cancerous sore on her foot had healed completely, the black spots had disappeared and she had regained some strength. She was able to resume her twice daily walks along the seaside. Her physician and oncologist did not see her following her initial evaluation for a period of one year. At one year she was examined. No cancer was found, the melanoma was gone, the foot completely healed and with considerable surprise the physician announced that she 'no longer has any cancer'. The family was informed that she had an extremely strong immune system. At the age of 95 she is enjoying walks with her friends and family although these are shorter than they used to be. She experiences no pain from her prior melanoma although she is weaker than she used to be. This could be due to her overcoming the effects of Parkinson's symptoms that arose as a side effect of several conflicting Alzheimer's medications that were mistakenly administered at the same time.

FOLLOW UP:

Current health status: deceased
Time since diagnosis: n/a
Months in remission: 8 months

Eight months after she was declared to be cancer free she died from complications arising from the progression of her Alzheimer's disease along with the complications arising from receiving conflicting medications. She was 95 years old.

CHAPTER NOTES:

1. Canadian Cancer Society. Canadian Cancer Statistics 2010. Supplementary Figures. http://www.cancer.ca/Canada-wide/About%20cancer/Cancer%20statistics/~/media/CCS/Canada%20wide/Files%20List/English%20files%20heading/PDF%20-%20Policy%20-%20Canadian%20Cancer%20Statistics%20-%20English/Supplementary%20web %20figures.ashx
2. Canadian Cancer Society. Canadian Cancer Encyclopedia, Melanoma of the skin. http://info.cancer.ca/cce-ecc/default.aspx?Lang=E&toc=46&cceid=922
3. Canadian Cancer Society. Canadian Cancer Encyclopedia, Survival statistics for melanoma. http://info.cancer.ca/cce-ecc/default.aspx?Lang=E&toc=46&cceid=922
4. Schaefer BA, Hoon LT, Burke DM, et al: Nutrition and Cancer: Salvestrol case studies. *J Orthomol Med*, 2007; 22: 177-182.

10.
PERITONEAL CANCER WITH METASTASES IN THE OVARIES

Peritoneal cancer is a rare form of cancer involving the peritoneum. This cancer is more commonly diagnosed in women and is very rarely diagnosed in men. It shares a great deal of similarity with ovarian epithelial cancer and is often treated with the same chemotherapy agents. Given the rarity of this cancer there are no incidence statistics for the United Kingdom. However, it is known that between 7 and 15% of women diagnosed with advanced ovarian cancer have peritoneal cancer.[1]

Peritoneal cancer is most commonly detected in women over the age of 50. There is little known about the causes of this disease. The disease is difficult to detect in the early stages and consequently is only staged at stage 3 and stage 4. Peritoneal cancer is also likely to recur due to the fact that it is often detected at such an advanced stage. Apparently the prognosis is best the longer an individual remains in remission,[2] which would appear to be medi-speak for, 'it is more likely to rain when it's raining'!

PRIMARY PERITONEAL CARCINOMA – STAGE 3[3]

Age at diagnosis:	57
Date of diagnosis:	May 2011
Sex:	female
Country of residence:	England
Salvestrol points per day:	6,000 points per day
Time from start of Salvestrol use to being told she was cancer free:	7 months
Time in remission with no evidence of cancer:	13 months

A 57-year old woman visited her physician three times due to discomfort and distension in her abdomen. Upon her third visit her physician made a thorough investigation as she was now suffering from a very swollen abdomen, loss of appetite and fatigue. A computerised tomography (CT) scan of the abdomen and pelvis and a subsequent biopsy led to a diagnosis of stage 3 peritoneal carcinoma, a rare and aggressive cancer, with metastases in the ovaries. Her CA125, a blood test that reflects the activity of ovarian or peritoneal cancer, was markedly elevated at 7,250.

Her doctor's opinion was that she had been in a high risk category for cancer due to the occurrence of abdominal cancers in her immediate family and this may have predisposed her to her current condition. She was told that her condition was treatable and the following plan of treatment was outlined for her. She was to be given: a course of three rounds of chemotherapy followed by a month's rest. The surgery would be done, which included a radical hysterectomy and removal of any apparent cancer. She would then be given another month of rest and this would be followed by another three rounds of chemotherapy.

The patient accepted her physician's recommendation and started an intravenously delivered course of paclitaxel (for three hours) followed by carboplatin (for one hour) every three weeks. Ondansetron was prescribed twice daily for two days following chemotherapy to manage nausea and vomiting; however, its use was intermittent due to its constipating side-effect.

Along with the onset of chemotherapy, she embarked on an alternative treatment plan under the direction of a homeopathic physician and a medical herbalist. She began to supplement her diet with Salvestrols taking three Salvestrol (2,000 point) capsules per day comprising a daily total of 6,000 Salvestrol points. In addition she took three astragalus capsules per day. The homeopathic remedies included: Lachesis (three times daily); Kali Phosphoricum (twice daily); Phosphoricum Acidum (twice daily for 3-5 days following chemotherapy); and Natrum Muriaticum (twice daily for 10 days following chemotherapy). Acupuncture was used between chemotherapy sessions to increase appetite and energy level. She had

PERITONEAL CANCER WITH METASTASES IN THE OVARIES

an ongoing practice of meditation and visualisation which was continued throughout and after treatment, and she maintained a positive attitude. In terms of dietary changes, she cut out coffee consumption, increased her consumption of fruits, vegetables and green tea, and reduced her consumption of meat. Exercise consisted of daily walks.

After starting her treatment she suffered from persistent side-effects common to paclitaxel/carboplatin chemotherapy, including: anaemia (a decrease in red blood cell count); neutropenia (a low number of neutrophils – white blood cells); thrombocytopenia (a low level of platelets in the blood); loss of appetite; tiredness; loss of energy; face reddening as if sun burnt; weakness in knees; trouble walking; dizziness; trouble sleeping; numbness in arms, hands and feet; cold feet; noticeable bruising; aching legs; abdominal pain; nausea; a candida infection in the mouth; and a loss of taste. These side-effects resulted in the need for three blood transfusions before the six chemotherapy sessions were completed. Although the side-effects were severe and numerous it was the loss of her thick, long, beautiful hair that caused her the most anguish.

She maintained her alternative therapies, dietary change and walks throughout her treatment course. One week after starting her chemotherapy and alternative therapies there was a significant reduction in her abdominal swelling. By week four her CA-125 level had dropped to 4,593. Her CA-125 level was measured the day she received her third course of chemotherapy (week seven from onset of treatments) and it had dropped to 510. Her physician noted that she had never seen such a huge fall in CA-125 levels in all her career and was quite taken aback by the results thus far.

During the twelfth week of treatment she received a blood transfusion and a hysterectomy. The surgeon reported that most of the cancer had been removed except for "sugar grain-like" residual cancer. The post-operative pathology report noted a very good response to the therapy that she had been receiving. Unfortunately, the operation also left her suffering from constant abdominal pains.

Three weeks after the surgery the CA-125 level had fallen further to 52 and the doses for the fifth and sixth chemotherapies were consequently reduced by 20%. By week 19 of her treatment, the CA-125 had fallen to within normal limits. Chemotherapy was completed during week 22, and the CA-125 level was measured as 15 (within normal limits) the week following. At week 25 the CA-125 had fallen to 13. A CT scan was performed during week 28 and during the 29th week after treatment onset. She was told that she was cancer free. Her three month follow up confirmed this with a CA-125 level of 11.

This woman experienced a dramatic reduction of abdominal swelling a week after starting chemotherapy and alternative therapies. She also experienced unexpectedly dramatic reductions in CA-125 levels by week seven and continual reductions in these levels until reaching normal limits during week 19. This is a very impressive response for stage 3 peritoneal cancer or stage 3 ovarian epithelial cancer. Given the similarities between peritoneal carcinoma and ovarian epithelial cancer they are typically treated in the same way. If we look at the clinical trial literature for her conventional treatment, surgery plus paclitaxel/carboplatin chemotherapy, we find quite a varied rate of complete response (defined as no sign of cancer pathology remaining). Vasey reports a 28% complete response rate for the 296 patients studied (there were 538 patients were enrolled in this arm of the study[4]). In a smaller trial, Neijt reports a complete response rate of 40% in the relevant arm of his trial for the 67 patients that they used for this analysis – 100 patients were enrolled in this arm of the study.[5] In a further trial, du Bois reports a complete response rate of 31% for the 99 patients that they used for this analysis – 397 were enrolled in this arm of the study.[6]

Adverse effects are the primary reason for people failing to complete a clinical trial. Such patients either die, are removed from the study by attending physicians, or they remove themselves. It can be argued that in calculations of complete response rate for an intervention, one should use the total number of eligible people enrolled in each arm of the study, otherwise these response rates are artificially inflated. If we do this the complete response rates in the paclitaxel/carboplatin studies described above fall to 15% (from 28%), 27% (from 40%), and 8% (from 31%). These are not impressive complete response rates, given that surgical debulking of the tumour was performed, but they provide a context for the physician's surprise at her rapid recovery. We also have to question whether it was reasonable to subject this woman to the debilitating side-effects that she endured for the full 22 weeks of her treatment given these complete response rates.

She maintains her alternative treatment plan, dietary change and lifestyle changes, although she has returned to coffee consumption. She benefits greatly from her daily practice of meditation and visualisation and is currently writing a book on her cancer experience along with producing a visualisation CD for cancer patients. Her hair is growing back and she enjoys the unexpected benefit of looking younger with short hair. She believes that Salvestrols, and the other facets of her alternative treatment plan, played a key role in her return to good health.

FOLLOW UP:

Current health status:	enjoying good health and remains cancer free according to her physicians
Time since diagnosis:	21 months
Months in remission:	13

She has now had 13 months of remission and feels great. She maintains her dietary change, her lifestyle change, and her Salvestrol supplementation to prevent recurrence. She continues to work on her book and DVD to document her experience with cancer in the hopes of helping others to achieve remission and a return to good health.

PERITONEAL CANCER WITH METASTASES IN THE OVARIES

This woman certainly experienced a dramatic and complete response to a very advanced case of ovarian and peritoneal cancer. She used a combination of an intensive conventional program involving chemotherapy (with all of its adverse effects) and surgery, also with significant adverse effects. Two major questions present themselves. The first is: (1) could she have experienced a similar result without conventional treatment at all? (2) will her response last indefinitely, as long as she continues Salvestrols and her current lifestyle program? Only time and the continuation of this program will give us the answer to this question.

It is not uncommon to get a complete response to a conventional treatment program for ovarian cancer, although this woman's response was quite dramatic. The problem is maintaining this response. People will often experience a recurrence of the cancer 1 to 3 years after achieving a complete response. So, the issue here is whether or not Salvestrols and life-style changes can result in an indefinite remission of the cancer. Although I suspect that this might occur, we will require much more time and more similar cases to be completely comfortable with this outcome.

CHAPTER NOTES:

1. Cancer Research UK. Primary Peritoneal Cancer. http://www.cancerresearchuk.org/cancer-help/about-cancer/cancer-questions/primary-peritoneal-carcinoma
2. Gynecological Cancer Foundation. Understanding Primary

Peritoneal Cancer. http://www.wcn.org/downloads/primary_peritoneal_brochure.pdf

3. Schaefer, B., Potter G., Wood R., Burke D. Cancer and Related Case Studies Involving Salvestrol and CYP1B1. *J Orthomol Med,* 2012; 27: 131-138.

4. Vasey PA, Jayson GC, Gordon A, et al: Phase III randomized trial of docetaxel-carboplatin versus paclitaxel-carboplatin as first-line chemotherapy for ovarian carcinoma. *J Natl Cancer Inst,* 2004; 96: 1682-1691.

5. Neijt JP, Engelholm SA, Tuxen MK, et al: Exploratory phase III study of paclitaxel and cisplatin versus paclitaxel and carboplatin in advanced ovarian cancer. *J Clin Oncol,* 2000; 18: 3084-3092.

6. du Bois A, Lück HJ, Meier W, et al : A randomized clinical trial of cisplatin/paclitaxel versus carboplatin/paclitaxel as first-line treatment of ovarian cancer. *J Natl Cancer Inst,* 2003; 95: 1320-1329.

11.
PROSTATE CANCER

The prostate is a gland involved in the production of seminal fluid. It surrounds part of the urethra and consequently urination symptoms (such as frequent urination, getting up during the night to urinate or discomfort during urination), especially in men over 50, will typically trigger an investigation to determine if the prostate gland is enlarged and compressing the urethra. An enlarged prostate may be caused by a benign inflammation of the prostate (prostatitis), a benign enlargement of the prostate (benign prostatic hypertrophy or BPH) or prostate cancer. Frequently, prostate cancer may be present without any symptoms whatsoever. A screening blood test, known at the prostate specific antigen or PSA, when elevated, may suggest the possible presence of prostate cancer. In Canada and in the US the cancer with the highest incidence in men is prostate cancer. In Canada the estimate for 2012 is 26,500 new cases of prostate cancer which represents 14% of all cancer diagnoses and 27% of all cancer diagnoses for men.[1]

Prostate cancer is most commonly diagnosed in men over the age of 65. It is typically slow growing and consequently one often hears that more men die with prostate cancer than from prostate cancer. The prostate is not a life sustaining organ of the human anatomy and consequently prostate cancer does not represent an immediate threat to life. It is metastases from prostate cancer that are of greater concern than the prostate cancer itself, as these can afflict vital organs such as the liver, the lungs or the brain. Bone metastases from the prostate can result in significant pain and morbidity. Given this it is hard to comprehend why a search for metastases is so seldomly conducted prior to embarking on a treatment plan for the prostate cancer. Nevertheless the five-year survival figures for prostate cancer are quite good in comparison to the cancers that directly affect life sustaining organs. In Canada those that have been diagnosed with prostate cancer have a 96% chance of being alive at the end of five years compared with those that have not had a cancer diagnosis.[2]

PROSTATE CANCER[3]

Date of diagnosis:	October, 2004
Age at diagnosis:	74
Sex:	male
Country of residence:	UK/Canada
Salvestrol points per day:	1133 points

*Time from start of
Salvestrol use to being
told he was cancer free:*   18 months
*Time in remission with
no evidence of cancer:*   82 months

A 74-year-old gentleman received a prostate-specific antigen (PSA) test result of 11 ng/ml in the blood during his annual check-up (normal is up to 5 in the UK depending on age – this normal range differs from country to country). His previous PSA result had been 4 ng/ml so he was referred to a specialist. The specialist stated, "You have a PSA of 11 and I suspect that you have cancer. If you have treatment would you rather have surgery or radiation?" The gentleman replied, "If you were in this chair, which would you rather have?" The specialist suggested radiation!

Follow-up magnetic resonance imaging (MRI) and full body X-ray confirmed a diagnosis of prostate cancer (no biopsy was done as a biopsy is not always deemed necessary for a prostate cancer diagnosis in the UK). Surgery and radiation were both subsequently ruled out by the specialist through discussion with the patient. The specialist suggested an injection of the synthetic hormone leuprolide acetate (Prostap®) every three months to treat the symptoms of the prostate cancer (leuprolide acetate is not considered to be curative with respect to prostate cancer). This drug results in the patient producing less testosterone and generally slows down the worsening of prostate cancer since testosterone generally enhances prostate cancer growth. The gentleman was advised that this treatment would be required for the rest of his life. No other drugs were prescribed.

Subsequently this gentleman spoke to his cousin, a university lecturer, who told him that one of his students had been diagnosed with a terminal cancer of the brain and after taking Salvestrols had proved to her doctors that 'terminal' seemed to be an overstatement. He decided to begin Salvestrol supplementation taking two (350 point) Salvestrol capsules per day. He began taking the Salvestrols concurrent with his anti-testosterone treatment which frequently results in significant adverse effects, such as loss of libido, inability to function sexually and enlargement of breasts.

Six months after receiving his diagnosis his PSA level had dropped to below 1 ng/ml – well within normal limits. However, during this time he suffered from breast development, complete loss of body hair, impotence and a complete lack of libido as a result of the synthetic hormones. He complained that he now made Dolly Parton look flat chested!

He moved from England to Canada necessitating a change of doctors. At the time of the move he switched Salvestrol products and began taking one (1,000 point) Salvestrol capsule per day and one (350 point) Salvestrol capsule three times per day. The new doctor continued to monitor him using the PSA test and maintained quarterly injections of Lupron® (a different brand of leuprolide acetate). Twelve months after receiving his diagnosis his PSA level had dropped to 0.2

ng/ml. Upon receiving a subsequent PSA test result the new physician said that the PSA level received was as low as it could be and asked if the patient was sure that he had not had surgery! Given the physician's surprise that such a result could be attributed to leuprolide acetate alone the patient confessed to taking Salvestrols. The physician then stated that he had a patient that he would like to start on Salvestrols and asked the patient to supply him with background information. The physician decided to 'wean' the patient off of the quarterly Lupron® injections. Four months later he received his final injection of Lupron®.

FOLLOW UP:

Current health status:	enjoying good health – cancer free
Time since diagnosis:	100 months
Months in remission:	82

This gentleman has not had a Lupron® injection for nearly seven years and continues to receive PSA test results at the 0.2 ng/ml level – well within normal limits. His physician assures him that he remains cancer free. He has continued to supplement his diet with Salvestrols and has embarked on a fitness program and change in diet towards more fruit and vegetable consumption. His only complaint is the length of time it takes for diminishment of the breast development brought on by the use of Lupron®.

PROSTATE CANCER[4]

Date of first diagnosis: May, 2003
Age at diagnosis: 69
Sex: male
Country of residence: Canada
Salvestrol points per day: 429 points
Time from start of
Salvestrol use to being
told he was cancer free: 3 months
Time in remission with
no evidence of cancer: 79 months

A 72-year-old male was diagnosed with prostate cancer for a second time as part of the routine monitoring of his prior condition. This gentleman has a long-held belief that pharmaceutical approaches to disease treatment should only be considered as a last resort and preferred to look towards nutrition and nutritional supplements to restore his health. He had been diagnosed with prostate cancer three years earlier, and had successfully treated this occurrence with a combination of exercise, good nutrition, lycopene and a pollen-based supplement known as Protaphil®. He was subsequently pronounced 'all clear' by his physician. After three years of remission his regular prostate specific antigen (PSA) test scores started to climb. To confirm a diagnosis of prostate cancer, uPM3™ [5], a urine-based genetic test for prostate cancer from Bostwich Laboratories, was ordered to test for presence of the PCA3 gene that is profusely expressed in prostate cancer tissue. The results were positive for prostate cancer.

For this second diagnosis his doctor recommended that he supplement his diet with Salvestrols. He combined Salvestrol supplementation with a variety of other nutritional supplements: vitamin C; Co-Q10; folic acid; garlic; lycopene; zinc; cranberries; 2 multivitamins without iron; and vitamin E. Unfortunately we are unable to verify the dosage of any of these supplements other than the Salvestrol. With breakfast on Monday, Wednesday and Friday this gentleman took one Salvestrol (1,000 point) capsule which equates to a daily intake of Salvestrol of 429 Salvestrol points.

After a period of three months, a further PSA test was conducted and the result was within normal limits. His urologist pronounced him 'all clear' for the second time. Upon receiving this news he reduced his Salvestrol intake to one Salvestrol (350 point) capsule per day with his breakfast. He continues to be active, physically and mentally. He has had four further PSA tests at three-month intervals and they have all shown results within normal limits. He is now monitored annually. This gentleman has successfully defeated cancer twice without recourse to surgery or treatments with known adverse side effects.

FOLLOW UP:

Current health status: *enjoying good health – cancer free*

Time since first diagnosis: 117 months
Months in remission: 79

This gentleman has maintained Salvestrol supplementation, good nutrition and maintains an active life mentally and physically. He has now remained in remission for over six and one half years. This is a much better outcome than he realised with his first diagnosis of cancer where he remained in remission for three years. He made a particularly dramatic recovery from his second cancer diagnosis in that he made a full recovery in three months with a very small daily intake of Salvestrols. Both of his instances of prostate cancer were overcome without recourse to surgery or treatments with known adverse side effects. Perhaps the fact that his body was not trying to cope with, or overcome the added strain of these more aggressive therapies contributed to his ability to respond so quickly to such a low daily intake of Salvestrol for this second diagnosis.

PROSTATE CANCER, GLEASON SCORE 6 (3+3)[4]

Date of first diagnosis: May, 2008
Age at diagnosis: 79
Sex: male
Country of residence: Canada
Salvestrol points per day: 5,000 points
Time from start of Salvestrol use to being told he was cancer free: 7 months

PROSTATE CANCER

*Time in remission with
no evidence of cancer:*   60 months

A 79-year-old man received two elevated PSA test results with one week between tests. A digital rectal examination (DRE) indicated the presence of a tumour on the left side of the prostate. He was referred to an urologist who scheduled a biopsy for confirmation. The biopsy confirmed a diagnosis of prostate cancer and a Gleason Score of 6 (3+3) was assigned (The Gleason Score is a means of grading prostate cancer on a scale of 0 – 10 with 10 being most advanced). A full body scan was also carried out and results indicated that no metastases could be found.

Upon receipt of the confirmed diagnosis, this gentleman began taking Salvestrols on a daily basis. He took five Salvestrol (1,000 point) capsules per day, with two taken in mid-afternoon and three taken near midnight (5,000 points per day). These were taken in concert with his previous, thorough and long-term daily supplementation of vitamins and minerals that included known Salvestrol co-factors such as biotin (625 mcg), niacin and niacinamide (1,145 mg), magnesium (606 mg), ascorbic acid (3,900 mg), and iron fumerate (20 mg). Vitamin D (800 I.U.), vitamin E (1,200 I.U.) and selenium (165 mcg) also formed part of the daily supplementation. No dietary changes were made and no change in exercise level was made. Prescription medications for diabetes, and ongoing heart and kidney conditions were maintained. In two months of supplementation the PSA test result indicated a level lower than that reported prior to his diagnosis.

A period of three months elapsed between receipt of his biopsy results and a consultation with his urologist. The urologist referred the gentleman to the British Columbia Cancer Agency. While he waited for his referral to an oncologist his PSA level fell by another 1.80 ng/ml to 5.50 ng/ml, down 2.80 ng/ml from the level at time of diagnosis. This drop in PSA level brought the PSA level to within normal limits for a man of this age in Canada[6]. Four months after receiving his diagnosis and starting his Salvestrol supplementation and after his PSA had fallen to within normal limits he was interviewed by an oncologist at the Agency. Although his PSA level was now within normal limits he was given the option of either hormone therapy or radiation treatment. He chose hormone therapy and immediately received an initial 10.8 mg injection of Zoladex® (goserelin) to help control the tumour growth along with a prescription for repeat injections every 12 weeks. Casodex® (bicalutamide), an antiandrogen, was also prescribed, 50 mg daily for twenty-one days.

A significant spike in PSA test results was found during the month following this injection. In the second month following this injection the PSA test results began to decline. During the following month the PSA test results indicated levels that led his oncologist, after carrying out a digital rectal examination, to suggest no further treatment as the cancer was said to be in remission. The gentleman was told that he would be followed every three months for one year then every four months for a further year. All injections and prescription drugs were stopped.

Upon receipt of this news the Salvestrol supplementation was reduced to two Salvestrol (1,000 point) capsules per day, with both taken in mid-afternoon (2,000 points per day). His PSA level had fallen to within normal limits before conventional treatment began. He received a single injection of Zoladex®, 10.8 mg, before being declared in remission by his oncologist. Zoladex® is an LHRH agonist intended for long term use, administered every 12 weeks[7]. This gentleman's experience suggests that for those individuals that utilise LHRH agonists, concurrent use of Salvestrols or other nutritional therapy may bring about a quicker response and diminish the need for further hormonal injections.

FOLLOW UP:

Current health status:	enjoying good health – cancer free
Time since diagnosis:	67 months
Months in remission:	60

This gentleman has now been in remission for five years. His PSA level had fallen to within normal limits before conventional treatment was started. After conventional treatment was finished he has maintained his Salvestrol supplementation and has enjoyed good health although he is now experiencing some age related health issues.

CHAPTER NOTES:

1. Canadian Cancer Society. Canadian Cancer Encyclopedia, Statistics for Prostate Cancer. http://info.cancer.ca/cce-ecc/default.aspx?toc=41
2. Canadian Cancer Society. Prostate Cancer Statistics at a Glance http://www.cancer.ca/Canada-wide/About%20cancer/Cancer%20statistics/Stats%20at%20a%20glance/Prostate%20cancer.aspx?sc_lang=en
3. Schaefer BA, Hoon LT, Burke DM, et al: Nutrition and Cancer: Salvestrol case studies. *J Orthomol Med*, 2007;22:177-182.
4. Schaefer BA, Dooner C, Burke DM, Potter GA. Nutrition and Cancer: Further Case Studies Involving Salvestrol. *J Orthomol Med*, 2010; 25, 1: 17-23.
5. Bostwick Laboratories Announces uPM3(TM) Test, First Genetic Test for Prostate Cancer. September 23, 2005. http://www.psa-rising.com/wiredbird/bostwick-labs92303.php
6. Canadian Cancer Society. Tests for Prostate Cancer http://www.cancer.ca/Canada-wide/Prevention/Getting%20checked/Tests%20for%20prostate%20cancer.aspx?sc_lang=EN
7. Product Monograph. Zoladex® 10.8 mg Goserelin/depot. Luteinizing Hormone – Releasing Hormone Analog (LHRH Analog). February 24, 2009. http://www.astrazeneca.ca/documents/ProductPortfolio/ZOLADEX%20LA_PM_en.pdf

12.
BENIGN PROSTATIC HYPERPLASIA

Benign prostatic hyperplasia (BPH) is an enlargement of the prostate that leads to a variety of unpleasant symptoms, many of which have to do with difficulties with urination. It is very rare in men under the age of 40 but as men age the incidence increases to the point that a vast majority of men at 80 years of age will have an enlarged prostate.

This instance of BPH, has been included to highlight the fact that Salvestrols may bring about health benefits beyond their role in combating cancer. BPH presents certain symptoms that are shared with those suffering from prostate cancer. This chapter indicates that relief of these symptoms can be achieved through the use of Salvestrols. Whether this is due to a known anti-inflammatory function of some Salvestrols, or whether there were indeed cancer cells present for this patient, or a combination of both, we cannot tell. Nevertheless, CYP1B1, the enzyme essential for the activation and anticancer efficacy of Salvestrols, could well have been involved because BPH cells, although neither a cancer nor a precursor of cancer, overexpress CYP1B1 relative to normal prostate[1]. Furthermore, in some men diagnosed with BPH their prostate also contains *prostatic intraepithelial neoplasia (*PIN) cells[2], which are a precursor of cancer and they also overexpress CYP1B1[1].

BENIGN PROSTATIC HYPERPLASIA[3]

Age at diagnosis: 50
Date of diagnosis: May, 2010
Sex: male
Country of residence: Canada
Salvestrol points per day: 675 points per day
Time from start of
Salvestrol use to
symptom free: 6 months

A 50-year-old male visited his physician after experiencing lower urinary tract symptoms including weak flow and nocturia (the need to urinate during the night). A digital rectal examination (DRE) revealed a significantly enlarged prostate. A prostate specific antigen (PSA) test was performed and the results were within normal limits. He was diagnosed with benign prostatic hyperplasia (BPH) and told that there were three medication options for control of this condition.

These would include a low dose alpha blocker (to relax smooth muscles in the prostate and neck of the bladder), followed by a higher dose alpha blocker if relief was not found. If relief was still not found a 5alpha-reductase inhibitor would be tried to try and slow the growth of the prostate. Whichever option produced relief would be required for life. This lifelong need for medication was very distressing to this fellow.

He was prescribed a low dose, 0.4 mg, of the alpha-adrenergic blocker, Flomax® (tamsulosin) to be taken once daily and asked to minimise his fluid intake after early evening. Initially he complied with moderating his fluid intake but quickly found this too difficult to maintain. No beneficial change was noted in the first week of Flomax® use. In the second week of use there was stronger urinary flow and diminished nocturia. These benefits lasted for two months at which time the benefits slowly diminished until by the end of his four month prescription little lasting benefit remained. Throughout the course of Flomax® treatment he experienced a low grade, dull headache upon waking in the morning. The headache subsided as the day progressed.

With the first prescription for Flomax® finished and knowing that the next treatment option was simply a higher dose he began looking for alternatives. After hearing anecdotal accounts of relief from BPH using Salvestrols he began taking one Salvestrol capsule (350 points) each morning. Within a month the incidence of nocturia had dropped down to once a night, sometimes not at all, and the flow was as strong as or stronger than it had been during the period when

Flomax® was working most effectively. After three months of Salvestrol supplementation he switched to a 1,000 point Salvestrol capsule. He reported that there was a noticeable improvement in terms of decreased incidence of nocturia and increased strength of flow. Although unable to quantify the improvement he noted that he no longer had to be as mindful of his evening fluid intake.

Concurrent with his use of Salvestrols for BPH he maintained his existing daily vitamin supplementation which included a multivitamin, a B-complex vitamin, vitamin C and vitamin D. No other dietary or lifestyle changes were made throughout this period. He enjoys a healthy, balanced diet that includes organic foods whenever practical to do so.

FOLLOW UP:

Current health status:	enjoying good health
Time since diagnosis:	28 months
Months in remission:	17

This fellow is still taking Salvestrol capsules, is enjoying a level of relief from BPH symptoms that is at least as good, if not better than that found when Flomax® was working most effectively and without the daily headaches that accompanied its use. Unlike Flomax®, the symptom relief found with Salvestrols has not diminished over time. Continual use of a food-based supplement such as Salvestrol does not cause him the distress that he felt when faced with the prospect of continual use of a prescription drug. Further cases will be needed to gain insight into the role of Salvestrols with benign prostatic hyperplasia.

CHAPTER NOTES:

1. Carnell DM, Smith RE, Daley FM, et al. (2004) Target Validation of Cytochrome P450 CYP1B1 in Prostate Carcinoma with Protein Expression in Associated Hyperplastic and Premalignant Tissue. *International Journal of Radiation Oncology Biology and Physics* 58: 500-509.
2. Vosianov AF, Romanenko AM, Zabarko LB, et al. (1999) Prostatic Intraepithelial Neoplasia and Apoptosis in Benign Prostatic Hyperplasia Before and After the Chernobyl Accident in Ukraine. *Pathology Oncology Research* 5: 28-31.
3. Schaefer, B., Potter G., Wood R., Burke D. Cancer and Related Case Studies Involving Salvestrol and CYP1B1. *J Orthomol Med,* 2012; 27: 131-138.

13.
STUDY FOLLOW UP

Over the years the people described in the previous chapters along with many others have used Salvestrols to help manage and overcome their cancer. As you have seen, these individuals represent a wide cross section of cancers, and all of these people have achieved remission. Over the last year I have been conducting a follow up on these people to get a sense of what factors have played a role in their remaining in remission or experiencing a recurrence. I have also undertaken a review of these situations to see if any further lessons could be learned. In this chapter I would like to review this data with you.

From the perspective of this dietary rescue mechanism, we do not view these people's recoveries as medical interventions – they represent situations in which long term dietary deficiencies of Salvestrol have been addressed. By way of introduction to this data, it is important to point out that we believe that when there has been a long term dietary deficiency resulting in a cancer diagnosis, an individual would most likely need a daily intake of between 4,000 to 6,000 Salvestrol points per day to overcome this deficiency and return to good health. An individual that has returned to good health after overcoming a cancer diagnosis would likely need a daily intake of 2,000 Salvestrol points per day to maintain their good health.

STUDY OVERVIEW

Table 1 provides a summary of the data from the cancer journeys described in the previous chapters.

The data points out that this dietary rescue mechanism does appear to have benefit across a broad array of cancers. The high incidence cancers are here: breast, prostate, lung, digestive tract along with an assortment of lower incidence cancers such as Hodgkin lymphoma, peritoneal, etc. You can also see that many of these situations represent people that did not receive conventional medical treatment while others received surgery, chemotherapy, radiation or some combination. The data covers males and females and an age range from 36 to 94 years of age. This overview also points out that there is quite a range in time taken to reach the all clear – 1 month to 18 months and also a range of daily Salvestrol intake to reach the all clear – 429 points to 6,000 points per day. Not everyone responds in the same way and not everyone carries the same tumour load.

Cancer diagnosis	Age	Sex	Points*	Surgery	Chemo	Radiation	Months to remission
breast	36	F	1975	N	Y	N	5
breast	50	F	2625	Y		Y	8
breast	76	F	1400	N	N	N	1
prostate	74	M	1133	N	Y	N	18
prostate	69	M	429	N	N	N	3
prostate	79	M	5000	N	Y	N	7
BPH	50	M	675	N	n/a	n/a	6
anal	46	M	1000	N	N	N	3
bladder	55	M	4000	Y	N	N	5
bladder, pancreas	61	M	4000	Y	Y	N	6
colon	64	F	3150	N	N	N	3
lung	69	M	4200	Y	N	N	1.5
liver	73	M	2864	Y	N	N	11
Hodgkin lymphoma	66	M	4000	N	Y	N	1.25
CLL	80	F	2000	N	N	N	3
melanoma	94	F	2917	N	N	N	12
peritoneal	57	F	6000	Y	Y	N	7

Table 1. Study Overview.

* indicates average Salvestrol points taken per day.

STUDY FOLLOW UP

RAPID RESPONDERS

Cancer diagnosis	Age	Sex	Points*	Surgery	Chemo	Radiation	Months to remission
breast	76	F	1400	N	N	N	1
Hodgkin lymphoma	66	M	4000	N	Y	N	1.25
lung	69	M	4200	Y	N	N	1.5
colon	64	F	3150	N	N	N	3
prostate	69	M	429	N	N	N	3
anal	46	M	1000	N	N	N	3

Table 2. Rapid responders.

This group is what I refer to as the rapid responders. The time taken to reach cancer free status (remission) ranges from 1 month to 3 months. I think that this is particularly interesting when we look at how little use of conventional medicine is represented in this group. In my opinion, the surgical intervention for the lung cancer patient was completely unnecessary. The tumours were shrinking so quickly and dramatically that if they had waited another 2 weeks it is altogether reasonable to assume that the tumours would have been entirely gone. At diagnosis he was told there was nothing that they could do for him as the size and placement of his tumour rendered him inoperable. Six weeks later they removed a small remnant of the tumour. This result was accomplished without the use of chemotherapy or radiation. He simply addressed the dietary deficiency through Salvestrol intake and dietary change. For the fellow with Hodgkin lymphoma, chemotherapy had been tried and failed prior to his commencement of Salvestrols. Certainly, not everyone responds this quickly, and one of the gentlemen in our array of studies took 18 months to achieve remission.

LOW SALVESTROL INTAKE RESPONDERS

Cancer diagnosis	Age	Sex	Points*	Surgery	Chemo	Radiation	Months to remission
prostate	69	M	429	N	N	N	3
anal	46	M	1000	N	N	N	3
prostate	74	M	1133	N	Y	N	18
breast	76	F	1400	N	N	N	1
breast	36	F	1975	N	Y	N	5
anal	46	M	1000	N	N	N	3
CLL	80	F	2000	N	N	N	3

Table 3. Low Salvestrol intake responders.

This group is interesting in that they have achieved cancer free status at very low daily intakes of Salvestrol. The average daily intake for these individuals ranges from 429 points per day to 2,000 points per day. Again as a group there is very little use of conventional medicine. They are making exceptionally efficient use of this Salvestrol/CYP1B1 rescue mechanism.

STUDY FOLLOW UP

RAPID RESPONSE AT LOW DAILY SALVESTROL INTAKE

Cancer diagnosis	Age	Sex	Points*	Surgery	Chemo	Radiation	Months to remission
prostate	69	M	429	N	N	N	3
breast	76	F	1400	N	N	N	1
anal	46	M	1000	N	N	N	3
CLL	80	F	2000	N	N	N	3

Table 4. Rapid response at low daily Salvestrol intake.

This group represents the response that we would like to see all the time. They achieve remission in three months or less at low daily intake of Salvestrol – 2,000 Salvestrol points or less per day. This is a group of individuals that we need to study in more detail, however, the current data point out some interesting aspects of this group.

None of these people had any conventional medical treatment. Half of them engaged in both dietary change (organic foods) and lifestyle changes, and three quarters of them engaged in dietary change. The woman with breast cancer made no changes. I think that these people represent what is possible when everything is working optimally. Their bodies are not trying to recover from the effects of surgery, chemotherapy or radiation. They seem to have excellent absorption of the Salvestrols, transportation of the Salvestrols, entry of the Salvestrols into the cancer cells and metabolism by CYP1B1. These people are likely getting from their diet or supplementation adequate levels of the Salvestrol co-factors that assist with efficient functioning of CYP1B1: iron, niacin, magnesium, vitamin C and biotin.

What I come away with from reviewing this group in particular, along with the rapid response group and the low dose response group, is that as soon as a lump is detected or a diagnosis is made, a person should immediately start to make dietary changes, lifestyle changes and start to take Salvestrols at recommended levels. If they do this, they may well be on the road to recovery or fully recovered before more aggressive procedures such as chemotherapy, radiation and surgery are scheduled. This could substantially reduce the risks to them from these more aggressive interventions and lead to a recovery free from debilitating side effects.

REMISSION FOLLOW UP

Cancer diagnosis	Age	Sex	Months in remission	Months in diagnosis	Status	Continued Salvestrols	Diet change	Lifestyle change
melanoma	94	F	8	n/a	deceased	Y	Y	N
breast	36	F	27	n/a	deceased	YN*	?**	?
prostate	69	M	79	117	remission	Y	Y	Y
prostate	74	M	82	100	remission	Y	Y	Y
breast	50	F	65	72	remission	N	Y	Y
colon	64	F	69	72	remission	Y	N	N
prostate	79	M	60	67	remission	Y	N	N

STUDY FOLLOW UP

anal	46	M	41	194	remission	Y	Y	Y
CLL	80	F	22	28	remission	Y	Y	Y
peritoneal	57	F	13	21	remission	Y	Y	Y
bladder, pancreas	61	M	16	32	remission	Y	N	N
BPH	50	M	17	28	remission	Y	N	N
lung	69	M	59	72	reccurent	N	N	N
bladder	55	M	19	152	reccurent	N	N	N
liver	73	M	36	76	reccurent	N	N	N
Hodgkin lymphoma	66	M	52	70	reccurent	N	N	N
breast	76	F	60	65	reccurent	YN	N	N

Table 5. Remission follow up.

YN* – finished using remaining Salvestrols on hand then stopped use

?** – unknown

Here we take a look at what happened after achieving remission. Two of the people studied have died. The older woman with melanoma died from complications arising from her Alzheimer's medication eight months after achieving remission. We do not know the cause of death for the young woman with breast cancer but a recurrent cancer would be a reasonable guess. It is always the best course to leave a family time to come to grips with their loss rather than to press them for follow up data.

We have a number of people that have a recurrence.

Some of these people remained in remission for quite some time, (e.g., five years). *One thing that binds this group together is that they all abandoned Salvestrol use and did not engage in dietary change or lifestyle change after being given the all clear.* It is difficult to make dietary and lifestyle changes. Of course a cancer diagnosis is highly motivating, but in the absence of that diagnosis, it is very easy to resort to prior habits.

We have a larger number of people that are still in remission. *What binds this group together is that all but one have continued taking Salvestrols.* The one woman that has not carried on with Salvestrols I am not worried about. She eats a strictly organic diet, she takes daily exercise and has an active yoga practice. If you met her you would think she was in her early 40s but in fact she is getting closer to 60. If you meet her for lunch or dinner she will kindly suggest restaurants that use only organically grown foods.

Taken together I think that this follow up data provides further support for the Professors hypothesis that CYP1B1 is a dietary rescue mechanism. When the diet has been deficient in Salvestrols over a long period of time and a cancer diagnosis is made, the individual can return to good health by addressing this dietary deficiency with sufficient daily intake of Salvestrols. The Salvestrol/CYP1B1 rescue mechanism will rid the body of the cancer cells. Once a person has achieved remission, they can enjoy good health over a long period of time by continuing with their dietary change, their lifestyle change, and their daily intake of adequate amounts of Salvestrol. The

Salvestrol/CYP1B1 rescue mechanism will continue to work on their behalf long after remission has been achieved. After all, remission means nothing other than no one is able to see or detect the presence of cancer – it does not necessarily mean the individual is cancer free. In addition, remission does not mean that the root cause of the cancer has been addressed, it only means that the visible manifestation of that cause, the tumour(s), have been dealt with. Given this, it is very important that people are informed of the benefits of long term use of Salvestrols, dietary change, and lifestyle change if they wish to remain cancer free.

LENGTH OF TIME IN REMISSION

Cancer diagnosis	Age	Sex	Months in remission	Months in dignosis	Status
breast	36	F	27	n/a	deceased
melanoma	94	F	8	n/a	deceased
prostate	74	M	82	100	remission
prostate	69	M	79	117	remission
colon	64	F	69	72	remission
breast	50	F	65	72	remission
prostate	79	M	60	67	remission
anal	46	M	41	194	remission
CLL	80	F	22	28	remission
BPH	50	M	17	28	remission
bladder, pancreas	61	M	16	32	remission

peritoneal	57	F	13	21	remission
breast	76	F	60	65	reccurent
lung	69	M	59	72	reccurent
Hodgkin lymphoma	66	M	52	70	reccurent
liver	73	M	36	76	reccurent
bladder	55	M	19	152	reccurent

Table 6. Length of time in remission.

In follow up studies of cancer patients it is typical to look at how many have survived for five years following news of their remission. In this collection of cancer journeys, many of them are far too recently diagnosed to be able to do this for the entire set. However, we can take a look at those that were diagnosed at least five years ago and see how well they have been doing.

Of those that remain in remission we have six cases that were initially diagnosed over five years ago. Of these, five have been in remission for five years or more – one of them has been in remission for just under 7 years. The remaining individual in this subset has been in remission roughly 3 ½ years and the reason for the difference is that our investigation involved his second diagnosis. He commenced Salvestrol use less than four years ago so he is actually doing very well.

Of those that have suffered recurrence all five of them were diagnosed more than five years ago. This group has survived but is currently dealing with recurrent cancers, however, all but one remained in remission for three years or more. One remained in remission for five years. The one that remained in remission for only 1 year was subsequently diagnosed with kidney cancer. Given the proximity of this second diagnosis to his recurrent bladder cancer diagnosis, it is a reasonable assumption that the kidney tumour was likely present but overlooked when he began his Salvestrol intake for his recurrent bladder cancer. Even the fellow with liver cancer has done surprisingly well, given his concurrent cirrhosis of the liver, stomach ulcer, pulmonary tuberculosis, and his return to alcohol consumption. He is still alive over six years after his initial cancer diagnosis and has been in remission for three of those years.

Another approach to determining how well this set of individuals are doing is to look at those situations in which the individual was given a life expectancy or other prognostic statement and see how well they have done against this prevailing medical thought. We have six situations in which the individual was given a specific prognostic statement. The fellow with papillary urothelial carcinoma, kidney cancer, and pancreatic cancer was told that he had a life expectancy between 2.5 and 5 months. He is still alive and cancer free 32 months after diagnosis. The woman with chronic lymphocytic leukaemia was given a life expectancy of between two days and 2 years. She is alive and cancer free 28 months after receiving her diagnosis and has been in remission for 22 months. The elderly woman with stage 4 melanoma was given a life expectancy of two weeks. She lived for 20 months after her diagnosis, 8 of those months in remission and subsequently died of complications arising from her Alzheimer's medications. The fellow with stage 3B Hodgkin lymphoma was told that he had one to two years to live. He is still alive 70 months after his diagnosis and has spent 52 of those months in remission. The man with stage 2-3 lung cancer was given 8 to 18 months to live. He is still alive 79 months after his diagnosis and has spent 59 of those months in remission. Finally the fellow with anal carcinoma was told that he had three years before an abdominoperineal resection necessitating a permanent colostomy would be required. He has managed to avoid this unpleasant prognosis for 189 months and has enjoyed 36 months of remission. Physicians do not provide these prognostic statements lightly. They provide them after assessing the various threats to the individual's health and existence. Beating these prognostic statements and beating them soundly provides further evidence that the Salvestrol/CYP1B1 rescue mechanism is a fundamental mechanism for achieving good health. When a diet deficient in Salvestrols is addressed, especially through switching to organic foods and supplementing with Salvestrols, this mechanism can greatly assist in beating the odds provided by prevailing medical thought.

Since many of the people described here were initially diagnosed less than five years ago we will continue our dialogue with them so that we can follow their progress past the five year mark and beyond.

STUDY FOLLOW UP

WHAT ABOUT THOSE THAT RESPOND VERY SLOWLY?

We have taken a look at situations where people have responded exceptionally quickly and at situations where people have responded at very low doses. These situations are great to look at and they show how people can return to good health when everything is working optimally. However, there are also people that respond slowly or feel that they are not responding at all. There can be many reasons for this. Certainly one of the reasons is that people often do not look to dietary change and nutritional approaches until they have availed themselves of all that conventional medicine has to offer and still found that the disease is advancing. In these situations the individual is very ill, the body is not working optimally and there is very little time for any approach to return the person to good health.

In order to understand what can be going wrong when someone is not responding in a reasonable time frame we first have to look at what happens when we ingest Salvestrols, either through our food or in supplement form. The Salvestrols have to be absorbed and be transported to the cancer cells (that is, they have to be bioavailable). They then have to enter the cancer cell and be metabolised by CYP1B1 to produce a metabolite that will initiate apoptosis. As you can see there are a variety of things that all must happen for the desired outcome. With a person in poor health all of these things are possible processes where a failure can occur.

When I hear that someone is having a poor response my immediate thought is that there may have been some exposure to CYP1B1 inhibitors (inhibitors prevent CYP1B1 from metabolising Salvestrols). Laetrile and supplement level doses of resveratrol will certainly inhibit CYP1B1 and thereby nullify any beneficial effect of taking Salvestrols. Outside of these inhibitors there are a host of environmental inhibitors of CYP1B1, mainly in the form of fungicides. One can encounter fungicidal inhibitors of CYP1B1 on farms, golf courses, public gardens and also in a host of products. Paint, carpeting, dandruff shampoo, heating vent cleaners, new cars, etc., can all contain fungicides that can inhibit CYP1B1. Herbicides that contain glyphosate are also potent inhibitors of CYP enzymes. Residues can be found on many commercially grown crops. In light of this a systematic look for sources of CYP1B1 inhibition is a very good idea in these situations.

A further problem can occur when one is deficient in certain vitamins and minerals such as magnesium, niacin, biotin, vitamin C or iron. All of these are important co-factors for the proper and efficient functioning of CYP1B1. Deficiency in any one of them can seriously impair the ability of CYP1B1 to efficiently carry out its functions. This problem can be overcome by incorporating a good multivitamin that contains the vitamins and/or minerals that you are deficient in, into one's daily routine.

We also need to consider whether or not the Salvestrols are being absorbed and transported so that they can reach the cancer cells. In the gut the plant sugars need to be removed before the more hydrophilic Salvestrols can be absorbed. If one has taken many antibiotics there may not be a healthy enough mix of gut flora to remove these plant sugars as it is the gut flora (bacteria) that performs this function. Without absorption no beneficial effect will be realised. This situation can be remedied with a broad spectrum probiotic.

Once absorbed the Salvestrols then need to be readied for transit through the body. For the more hydrophilic Salvestrols a human sugar needs to be attached in order for them to be transportable. This function takes place in the liver and depends on good liver function. It is important to have your physician monitor your liver function to ensure that you are making beneficial plant nutrients bioavailable through the addition of a human sugar. For the more lipophilic Salvestrols a good mix of unrefined fatty acids will assist with their transportation especially when the target cancer is in the brain. A good mix of unrefined fatty acids can assist with transportation across the blood brain barrier.

A further difficulty can result from concurrent fungal infection. It is quite common for people to have significant fungal infections concurrent with their cancer diagnosis. In this situation any Salvestrols that are ingested, either in the form of food or supplements, will be utilised in combating both the fungal infection and cancer. It stands to reason that this is a situation where progress in dealing with the cancer diagnosis will be slower unless a much higher dose of Salvestrols is used that can bring about good progress on both the fungal infection and the cancer.

With the issues of CYP1B1 inhibition, operational efficiency due to vitamin and mineral deficiencies, absorption of Salvestrols and transportation of Salvestrols in good shape we need to ensure that the kidneys are working appropriately for ridding the body of waste material brought about by the CYP1B1/Salvestrol mechanism killing the cancer cells. When the body does not efficiently remove this waste infection can result which can set recovery back. It is important to have your physicians ensure that your kidney function is up to the task of clearing cellular debris so that this debris can be eliminated.

With these issues under control one also needs to consider the state of mind. A cancer diagnosis can bring about a massive amount of stress. This level of stress can be further heightened through the failure of various therapeutic interventions. It can be heightened further still through physician comments such as 'is your will in order'! For decades the deleterious effect of stress on health has been studied. Stress will not help you recover. Fortunately in the past decade there has been a growing body of research looking not at a stress response but at a relaxation response, for lack of better phraseology. This research shows that through a brief daily practice of yoga, meditation, breathing exercise and/or visualisation gene expression can be altered in ways that are beneficial for health recovery. Almost everyone fighting a serious illness suffers from stress. Check your state of stress and how much of the day is spent enduring this stress and seek resources that will teach you a simple yoga routine or a simple meditation or visualisation routine that you can quickly and easily incorporate into your daily routine. This will not only help to moderate the deleterious effect of the stress, it will also start to bring about beneficial physiological change towards health recovery and the bonus is that you will probably really enjoy it.

Finally, when you are feeling like your recovery is moving too slow and you have worked through all of the above remember our gentleman with prostate cancer that took 18 months before he was told he was clear of the disease. At time of writing he has now been clear of this disease with no recurrence for 7 years!

SUMMARY:

- Check for exposure to CYP1B1 inhibitors and avoid: laetrile, resveratrol, fungicides, herbicides.
- Check for deficiency in magnesium, niacin and iron. Remedy with a good multivitamin.
- Check the state of gut flora. Remedy with a broad spectrum probiotic.
- Check liver function for making plant nutrients bioavailable. Remedy with liver function tests followed by physician's recommendations.
- Check the dietary mix for fatty acids. Remedy is to increase dietary intake of unrefined

fatty acids and or supplement the diet with unrefined fatty acids.
- Check for concurrent fungal infection. Remedy with a higher dose of Salvestrols if present.
- Check elimination of cellular debris from cancer cell death. Remedy with kidney function tests followed by physician's recommendations.
- Check stress levels. Remedy this with daily yoga, meditation and/or visualisation.
- Don't succumb to discouragement. Remedy this with the knowledge that the disease took many, many years to develop and may take many, many months to resolve.

WHAT DID WE LEARN FROM THE FOLLOW UP?

The follow up of these individuals has pointed to three central conclusions.
- *First:* The Salvestrol/CYP1B1 rescue mechanism works across a very broad array of cancers, providing further evidence that this is a truly universal mechanism for the protection of and restoration of our health. These situations provide further, real-world evidence, that cancer is a dietary deficiency.
- *Second:* The Salvestrol/CYP1B1 rescue mechanism should be activated at the earliest opportunity, as soon as a lump is detected or a cancer suspected. An immediate switch to a diet rich in organic fruits and vegetables,

some light daily exercise and an intake of between 4,000 and 6,000 Salvestrol points per day through supplementation could result in remission being achieved before aggressive treatments are initiated. This could lead to a side effect free journey from illness to good health. Better still you should activate this rescue mechanism preventatively so as to help avoid a diagnosis.

- *Third:* It is especially important that the Salvestrol/CYP1B1 rescue mechanism continue to be activated through continued dietary change (organic fruit and vegetable consumption), modest daily exercise, and daily intake of 2,000 Salvestrol points through supplementation, if remission is to remain over the long term. Remission does not mean that the cause of the cancer has been addressed and it does not mean that you are cancer free. If this dietary rescue mechanism has returned you to good health, ensure that you keep utilising it so that it can maintain your good health over the rest of your life.

14.
WHEN ARE WE WELL?

OVARIAN CANCER, STAGE 3

Diagnosis:	ovarian cancer
Date of first diagnosis	
(stage 2 ovarian cancer):	October 2006
Date of second diagnosis	
(stage 2 ovarian cancer):	August 2009
Date of third diagnosis	
(stage 3 ovarian cancer):	October 2010
Age at first diagnosis:	52
Sex:	female
Country of residence:	South Africa
Salvestrol points per day:	variable – 4,000 points for 12 months, then 8,000 points for 2 weeks, then 12,000 points for a few months then back to 8,000 points which is currently being taken

Time from start of
Salvestrol use to
cancer free: not applicable
Time in remission: not applicable

The people that we have the pleasure of working with teach us a great deal about overcoming disease. They educate us, encourage us, motivate us, and inspire us. From time to time one of them will not only teach us a great deal about overcoming disease but teach us about life itself. There is a woman that I have been working with for the past couple of years and I would like to present her situation, not to highlight recovery, per se, but rather because I think that her approach to her situation and life itself can be of benefit to others suffering with cancer.

She received her first diagnosis of stage 2 ovarian cancer in October 2006 at the age of 52. It was treated successfully using conventional medicine. In August 2009 she was diagnosed with her second diagnosis of stage 2 ovarian cancer. Again this was treated successfully using conventional medicine. In October 2010 she received her third diagnosis of transitional cell carcinoma of the ovary, this time it was stage 3 – transitional cell carcinoma is a rare subtype of ovarian surface epithelial cancer. Elevated levels of the cancer marker CA125 led to a referral to medical imaging. Medical imaging revealed two tumours near the pelvic wall and tumours in two of her lymph nodes. Biopsies confirmed a diagnosis of recurrent cancer. She was told that two of the four tumours could be removed through an extensive and risky surgical procedure while two could not be removed. She was also told that her condition could be controlled with chemotherapy but not cured. This news was very upsetting to her. She had been dealing with cancer for four years and no one had told her that her cancer was not curable. She decided to decline the surgery and the chemotherapy and search for ways of dealing with the cancer on her own. Fortunately her daughter-in-law was a nutritionist and provided her with recommendations for dietary change and supplementation that included Salvestrols.

At the end of one year of Salvestrol supplementation, further nutritional supplementation, and dietary change her CA125 levels had dropped to a level just outside the normal range. She reported that she felt 'a thousand times better than before the cancer made its reappearance. She also reported that her skin was clear and symptoms related to her osteo-arthritis had all but cleared up.

Just after this one year mark her CA125 level doubled. She doubled her daily intake of Salvestrols, added liposomal vitamin C, liposomal glutathione and a probiotic to her daily wellness plan. One month later her CA 125 fell by about 25%. During the following month her CA125 level shot up well past the level it had reached when it doubled. She was sent for more blood tests and imaging. After a further two months she saw her oncologist. Her CA125 level had fallen somewhat and she was told that medical imaging revealed that two of the tumours were now not visible but there appeared to be one tumour where there had been two previously and the size of this single tumour was slightly larger than the two previous tumours combined. Her oncologist told her that she had never seen anyone do so well without the benefit of chemotherapy. There were no signs of further metastases and all of her vital organs appeared to be working well.

During this time I was in routine contact with her. She is a very cheery person but upon returning from her medical appointments she would invariably be distressed by the unpredictable movements of her cancer marker CA125. She also knew that no curative solution was available from conventional medicine. She would remain distraught for a few days and then return to her cheery self until the next visit to the doctor. She carried on like this for another couple of months and her CA125 levels continued to disappoint her. At this point she took a bit of a reassessment. Fortunately, during this entire third diagnosis, she had no symptoms and no pain. However, when your cancer marker is well outside the normal range, your physician is concerned, as is everyone that hears the news. Consequently, the cancer sufferer in turn feels concern and this concern can translate into depression and a feeling of hopelessness.

She began to think that these feelings of distress and anguish following her medical appointments were at odds with who she was. She felt that she could no longer base her own assessment of how she was doing on this cancer marker, as all it appeared to do was confuse and depress her. So she decided to simply base her assessment of her own health on how well she felt and she felt great! She decided that she would continue to be monitored by her physicians, but on a day by day basis, she would conduct herself and make decisions about her life according to how well she felt rather than how she thought she should feel based on a cancer marker result or imaging results.

From the strength of this perspective she empowered herself – people that are well can do things and enjoy life!!! She took a course at the local college, a course in a healing modality, and began volunteering at a senior's facility so that she could use her new skill to benefit the residents. She also took a five week holiday in India. Upon returning from India she promptly booked a three week trip to Australia with her grandson so that the two of them could visit her daughter. She meets each day with enthusiasm and optimism, and I can certainly say from my own interactions with her that she extends her cheeriness and enthusiasm to all that she encounters. She now lives in sync with the person that she is rather than in sync with the person that her medical results say she is.

Does she want to have a CA125 level that is within normal limits and stays there? Yes, she would dearly like this but she says that until then she chooses to live her life from the perspective of, 'I am healed when I feel like I'm healed'. Since she feels great she lives her life without limitations and fear and consequently gets a great deal of joy out of life, and those around her get a great deal of joy out of their interactions with her.

Does she have a good approach? She has used no conventional treatment, since none would actually cure her, and she is currently feeling great 29 months after her third cancer diagnosis. She remains an inspiration to the whole team. She has transformed her life with a single, compelling thought!

FOLLOW UP:

Current health status:	enjoying good health – symptom free
Time since first diagnosis:	77 months
Time since third diagnosis:	29 months
Months in remission:	not applicable

About a month and a half ago she was scheduled for more medical imaging and an appointment with her oncologist. The CA125 level had risen over 500 and medical imaging revealed that the single tumour was now larger (9 cm) and pressing on both the bladder and rectum. Although the tumour did not appear to have invaded either, the oncologist recommended surgery to remove it. The oncologist added that she *"was in the very blessed 10% to still be so well and that she has NEVER had a patient be in this good condition after NO chemo or other treatment – she said typically she expected to see a huge spread [of the cancer] and there is NONE !"*

Two surgeons performed the surgery. The tumour was much deeper than they anticipated and firmly attached to the colon/rectum. In order to spare her from a permanent colostomy they removed what could be removed without damaging the colon/rectum. This meant leaving a layer of aberrant plaque like cells attached to the wall of the colon/rectum. The most interesting facet of the surgery was that the tumour was a soft, cyst like tumour, consisting mainly of fluid in a shell-like casing with a plaque like outer layer. This tumour description points to the difficulty in determining what is actually going on when one has only medical imaging and existing tumour markers to go on. Although the mass was distinctly bigger than previous, this growth did not appear to be the result of tumour growth but rather from fluid buildup within the confines of the tumour encapsulation. This is a much better situation than the one anticipated when surgery was recommended and indicates that she has been on the right track with her wellness plan.

She has recovered very nicely from the surgery and is waiting for her follow up appointment with her oncologist. While waiting she has booked a flight to Canada with a departure in two months' time to take a week long course exploring consciousness that she has been wanting to take. When she arrives in Canada, my job will consist of making sure that she sees a bear in the wild while she is here!

15.
ONE LAST STORY

Years ago I had the good fortune of meeting Dr. Abram Hoffer. Abram was a medical doctor and biochemist who maintained clinical practice while pursuing research. He did great work in the area of nutrition and mental health and co-founded the International Society for Orthomolecular Medicine along with Dr. Linus Pauling.

Everyone that knew Abram realised that he had a personal story for almost every health related circumstance that could arise. My favourite of Abram's stories was told during a lunch discussion on the role of hope in recovery – how a change in perspective could change the course of one's recovery. The perfect story to follow from the previous story of the South African woman with ovarian cancer.

Dr. Hoffer mentioned that when he was working as a young intern in a hospital in New York, a man suffering from stage 4 cancer was admitted for palliative care. The man was dying and everyone knew it. After a few days in hospital the man was visited by an old friend. With great trepidation the old friend mentioned that the dying man's wife couldn't wait any longer for his demise and had moved her new boyfriend into their home. They were boxing up his belongings to ship off to a charity. The old friend was very sorry to pass this news along but couldn't leave it unsaid.

The dying man reflected on this shocking news overnight. In the morning he got dressed, checked himself out of the hospital and went home. Upon arriving at his home he promptly threw his wife and her new boyfriend out. With the house to himself he then turned his attention to disentangling himself from his wife. He unpacked his things from the boxes his wife and her boyfriend had put them in. He put his things away, and then gathered up her belongings, boxed them up, and got them delivered to her. He changed the locks on the house and went through all the various bits of paperwork to make sure that all facets of his life would be run by him and him alone – bills, taxes, etc. He consulted a lawyer and set to divorcing his wife. Three months into this disentanglement the paperwork was starting to fall into shape and it suddenly dawned on him that he no longer had an income! He had left his job when he was deemed too ill to work. He called up his prior employer, who was quite surprised to hear from him, and requested his old job back. His employer accepted him back without question (how do you say no to someone in his circumstance, eh?). A year later he had a minor ailment that caused him to visit his doctor. His doctor was extremely surprised that he was still alive and sent him for a full investigation for cancer. He was cancer free!

I don't advocate tossing your spouse out as a cure for cancer or any other disease. However, Abram's story is worth keeping in the back of your mind. We are always, even in our darkest moments, more than a disease diagnosis, more than a set of physical symptoms, more than a patient. If we can keep this in mind, then perhaps we will be better able to shift our attention away from being ill, or terminal, or any other label that has been provided, and turn our attention to hope, optimism, and a return to good health. In so doing, we will utilise the enormous power of the mind body connection to help us through those darkest moments. Hope, and perhaps good health, is only a thought away.

[A version of this story was originally published by Health Action Network Society. Schaefer, B., September 2009 *Abram Hoffer – A Memorial Celebration*. www.hans.org and is re-told here with their kind permission]

16.
THE NEED FOR BETTER DIAGNOSTICS

Receiving a diagnosis of cancer is obviously distressing. It is very often made more distressing by the fact that the disease is so often detected only after it has advanced to the point of generating symptoms. There is a distinct need for advancements in the early detection of cancer – detection at a stage where dietary change and lifestyle change are more than enough to reverse the disease and return the individual to good health.

Once diagnosed, the journey itself is distressing in that often the monitoring of disease progression provides ambiguous and confusing information. This is more than highlighted in the situation that the South African woman, that I described earlier, faced. One of the central difficulties is that the tools in use at present do not represent a clear and unambiguous measure of the cancer itself – they are only indirect measures and as such, come with an element of uncertainty. In addition, the monitoring of many cancers is not done very frequently because no tools exist that can be used inexpensively and routinely without causing further harm to the patient (one cannot continue to use radiation based imaging on a frequent basis with a patient without further harm to their health). Given this, there is a real need for advancements in the monitoring of disease progression – unambiguous measures of disease progression over time that provide a clear picture to both the physician and the patient as to whether or not the disease is advancing, staying the same or diminishing – that is what is needed in future cancer monitoring tools.

Once the individual has achieved remission, they are typically monitored on an annual basis. However, these same inadequate tools are used for this purpose. A further difficulty is that the individual can be lulled into a false sense of security simply by being told that they are 'cancer free' or 'all clear'. None of us are cancer free! Even the healthiest of us will still have cancer cells develop. An individual that has been through a cancer diagnosis and achieved remission needs to be very vigilant to ensure that the conditions that gave rise to the first cancer diagnosis are not contributing to a subsequent cancer. To protect the health of those in remission, we also need advances in cancer detection and monitoring. We need direct measures of the presence of cancer with an accuracy and level of detection that permits alerting the patient to a recurrence early enough that dietary change and lifestyle change will be more than enough to reverse the progress of the disease.

Just to emphasise what is meant by cancer free, I would like to show you a graph taken from a great article by Dan Burke titled the 'Silent Growth of Cancer'. For medical technology to detect the presence of cancer, there must be about 10^9 cancer cells present. To provide a context for this fact, 10^9 cancer cells would occupy a space about half the size of your smallest finger nail – roughly the size of a pea. When you have 10^{12} cancer cells in your body (roughly a litre of cells) you are likely dead. The area of cancer growth between 0 and 10^9 cells is the Silent Growth of Cancer because it is not possible to tell whether or not there is cancer present. The difficulty for people that have been successful in beating their cancer and have been told that they are 'all clear' is that no one knows where on this curve they actually are. Are they all clear because all of the cancer cells are gone or are they all clear because the cancer cells have been reduced in number to just below the threshold (10^9) for detecting them? This graph helps to point out that a cancer survivor needs to remain vigilant about dietary change and lifestyle change if they wish to remain below the cancer detection limit.

THE NEED FOR BETTER DIAGNOSTICS

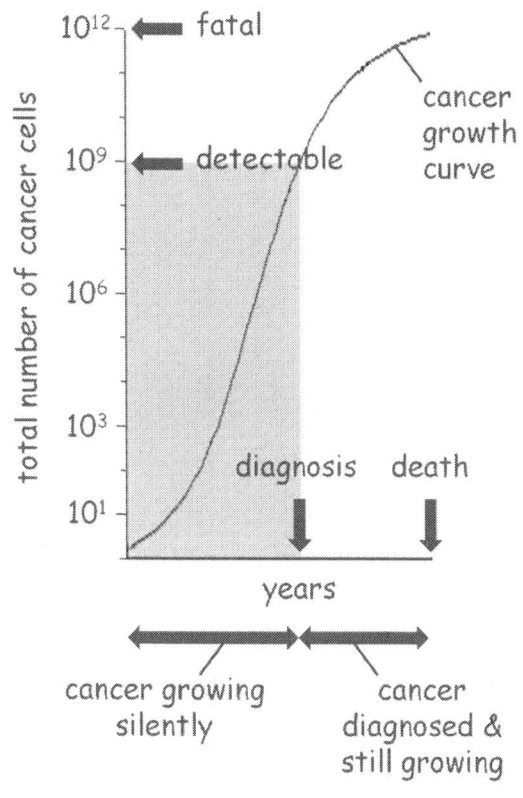

The Silent Growth of Cancer

This graph also highlights the earlier point that there is a real need for accurate tools for early cancer detection that can be delivered inexpensively. It also helps point to the need for accurate tools for cancer monitoring so that people have a real sense of progress made or lost so that their physicians can make better choices as to how to proceed.

Given this, we incorporated a company, CARE Biotechnologies, for the purpose of conducting research and development aimed at the realisation of tools for early cancer detection, cost-effective monitoring of disease progression, and accurate monitoring of those in remission. To achieve these aims we feel that we are in a great place to start from. We have a universal cancer marker in CYP1B1 and a vast amount of knowledge about this enzyme. We also know what CYP1B1 metabolises – Salvestrols and what their metabolites are and we have great expertise on these natural compounds. This provides us with a couple of unique possibilities for diagnostic development. We can either search for CYP1B1 itself, as a direct measure of the cancer or we can search for the metabolic output of CYP1B1, the metabolites, as a unique means of measuring the cancer.

METABOLITE TEST

Let's take a quick look at the metabolite test. To develop a test along these lines we first needed to examine a wide array of Salvestrols and their metabolites and find a metabolite that was not found in food and not produced by the metabolic activity of any other enzyme. That is, we needed a metabolite that was absolutely unique to a specific Salvestrol. With this we could then start to investigate the various ways in which we could take a sample of blood and prepare that sample so as to concentrate what we intended to look for while minimizing things that we did not want in the way. Sample preparation is really the key.

In this test what we want to find are two things: 1) the Salvestrol; and 2) its metabolite. Here is how this test works. A person is given a fixed amount of a specific Salvestrol. After a certain amount of time for the Salvestrol to be absorbed and dispersed, a sample of blood is taken. The blood is then prepared and analysed for the presence and quantity of the Salvestrol and the metabolite.

So let's contemplate three scenarios. In scenario 1 we find no Salvestrol but a big signal of metabolite. In scenario 2 we find a medium sized signal of Salvestrol and a medium sized signal of metabolite and in scenario 3 we find a big signal of Salvestrol and no metabolite signal. I know which scenario I would like to see – Scenario 3.

The scenario 3 result means is that the Salvestrols never got metabolised so this most likely means that the individual does not have cancer. If we already know that this individual has cancer then this result likely means that there is something interfering with the metabolic activity of CYP1B1.

In scenario 1 we know that this individual has cancer and enough cancer to fully metabolise all of the Salvestrol that was ingested. Although this is not good news, no one wants a cancer diagnosis, we can tell this individual that their cancer is metabolising Salvestrols very well. They would likely be wise to carry on taking Salvestrols and likely at a higher dose than they just ingested along with a switch to a diet high in organic fruits and vegetables. In short, we know that they have cancer and we know that the Salvestrol/CYP1B1 rescue mechanism will work efficiently.

In scenario 2 the individual also has cancer, and it is likely at a much lower stage of development than the person in scenario 1. Again we can tell this individual that their cancer is metabolising Salvestrols and they would be prudent to carry on taking Salvestrols at a level of daily intake such as that taken for the test or even at a lower amount. This person would also be wise to switch to a diet high in organic fruits and vegetables.

At the lab in England we have this test working and undergoing further refinement. What I really like about this test is that it uses natural products as diagnostics. Another nice feature of this test is that if we find the metabolite there isn't uncertainty – you have cancer and operational CYP1B1, so you are a good candidate for reversing the disease by addressing a dietary deficiency, that is, taking Salvestrols.

There is a lot that I like about this test. I especially like the ratio of Salvestrol measured to metabolite measured. I think that the more blood that we can analyse from people with confirmed cancer diagnoses the more we can fully understand the clinical implications of this ratio between Salvestrol levels and metabolite levels and this should translate into better prospects for cancer patients. Certainly our understanding can only improve, as work continues, with better clinical outcomes being the result.

THE NEED FOR BETTER DIAGNOSTICS

PROTEOMIC TEST

The other approach that we are taking is the proteomic test (the study of proteins). Rather than looking for the metabolic output of CYP1B1 in blood, we are looking for CYP1B1 itself. There are two primary ways in which CYP1B1 can end up in the blood. Enzymes have a short span of operation and the turnover of CYPs, such as CYP1B1, end up in the blood. The turnover of CYP1B1 is about three days. The second way in which the enzyme can end up in blood is through cancer cell death. Once killed the contents of the cell spill into the surrounding space and are ultimately absorbed into the blood. Of course a third, obvious way in which CYP1B1 can end up in blood is through blood based cancers – leukaemia.

By the time CYP1B1 reaches the blood, it can be partially broken down by various compounds so we don't actually look for the intact enzyme in the blood. What we do is look for a fragment of the enzyme that we know is unique to the enzyme and not forming part of any other human enzyme or any enzyme that could find its way into the human body through ingestion or bacterial infection.

To accomplish this, we raised an antibody, which is a protein that specifically binds to our fragment (peptide) and we use this antibody to help draw the peptide of interest out of the sample to concentrate the signal that we are looking for. Just like with the metabolite test, sample preparation is the key. We then use highly sensitive mass spectrometry equipment to analyse the sample for the presence and quantity of our peptide. When we find our peptide and measure its quantity, it provides us with a direct measurement of the cancer itself.

So far, this work has been progressing very well. We have a test operating that can detect our peptide in blood. In order to both calibrate the mass spectrometer and to provide a baseline with which to compare a cancer sufferer's blood, we analysed what is referred to as a proteomic standard. A proteomic standard is a sample of blood taken from a pool of blood drawn from a large number of healthy individuals. Everyone produces cancer cells on a daily basis, so even in the healthiest of individuals, there will be trace amounts of cancer, and in turn our peptide. Even at these trace amounts we were able to detect and measure the presence of our peptide in the proteomic standard. To make sense out of data that we received from analysing the blood of cancer sufferers, we assign a value of 1 to the amount of CYP1B1 in the proteomic standard. We then convert the values that we receive from the mass spectrometer into multiples of the amount found in the proteomic standard. When we analysed the blood of a sample of people suffering with lung cancer we found levels of CYP1B1 in their blood ranging from 93 times that found in the proteomic standard to 6291 times that found in the standard. We were very pleased with this result because the range suggests that we should be able to accurately assess each stage of cancer.

We are actively testing plasma from people with various cancers. We have found our peptide, that is, CYP1B1, in the plasma of people with colorectal cancer, ovarian cancer, lung cancer and most recently prostate cancer. To date the results have been highly encouraging. In addition, we have managed to get our test running on mass spectrometers that are more suited to use in commercial clinical laboratories, rather than just running on highly expensive research machines. We have also recently extended our research into developing assays (tests) for other CYP enzymes, such as CYP17, that we hope will further enhance the clinical picture provided by our CYP1B1 assay. Accurate monitoring of CYP17 levels is critical for clinicians using CYP17 inhibitors such as Zytiga® for control of prostate cancer. Prior to our development of this assay there was no efficient means of measuring these levels for ongoing monitoring of prostate cancer sufferers. We hope that we can provide this new CYP17 assay to clinicians within the next year to assist them in assessing treatment efficacy for their patients.

SUMMARY

I am very enthusiastic about both of these CYP1B1 tests and our new CYP17 test. The proteomic test provides us with exceptional sensitivity, enabling detection of disease at minute levels. If we can pick the disease up in a proteomic standard, then we can pick the disease up at a point where an individual has an excellent chance of reversing the disease with diet and lifestyle change alone. The metabolite test provides us with an excellent means of detecting the presence of cancer as well as reporting to us on the operational status of the CYP1B1 enzyme. With the metabolite test we can identify people that are most likely to have an excellent response to the use of Salvestrols. In terms of monitoring disease progression, both of these tests will be excellent. One of our goals with these tests is to get to the level of sensitivity and reliability that would enable us to tell whether or not a treatment is working within a matter of days.

Our research continues on both CYP1B1 tests alongside our research on the new CYP17 test. Further cancers will be tested, our methods will be refined, our approach will be extended to other CYP enzymes to enhance the clinical picture and we hope to soon be in a position to offer these tests to clinicians. Over the longer term, we feel that both of these approaches can be extended to other diseases. As soon as we have perfected our approach to cancer detection, we will turn our attention to development of diagnostics, based on these methods, to other diseases. We feel that the next few years will be exceptionally exciting for us because as we gather more and more data with our current blood tests, we will greatly expand our knowledge of how best to utilise Salvestrols and CYP1B1 for the benefit of those suffering from cancer.

17.
CONCLUSION

The people that are described here have all been through a very trying period of their life. They come from all over the world: Canada; England; New Zealand; South Africa; South Korea; and the United States, confirming the truly international extent of the suffering that this disease causes. They achieved remission and wanted to get on with the rest of their lives, but they took the time to work with us so that others could benefit from their experience, and we are very grateful to them. So what have we learned from their struggle?

For me the first lesson is that these people described here, and so many others that I have had the pleasure to meet, have met there darkest moments with an increased sense of compassion, kindness, humour and concern for others. This is what we are observing here through their revisiting of these painful times in the hopes that others will benefit. As we watch the evening news, we can often come away with a sense that humanity has lost its direction. These people, and so many others that face similar situations point to a different reality – a reality that renews our faith in humanity.

We have also certainly learned that cancer can be reversed through addressing a dietary deficiency. Bladder cancer, breast cancer, colon cancer, liver cancer, lung cancer, leukaemia, lymphoma, pancreatic cancer, peritoneal cancer, and prostate cancers all went into remission. This is exactly what one would expect from the research that confirms CYP1B1 as a universal cancer marker. Of these, we have six people that had no recourse to surgery, chemotherapy, or radiation therapy, and all of them managed to completely reverse the progress of their disease through Salvestrol supplementation and dietary change. This certainly supports the professors' hypothesis that the CYP1B1/Salvestrol mechanism is a rescue mechanism that utilises food-based compounds (Salvestrols) to rid the body of aberrant cells. It also shows us that there is a need to inform more medical doctors of the utility of incorporating nutritional approaches for cancer prevention, cancer management, and cancer treatment. The more medical doctors that study and embrace nutritional approaches, the better they will be able to care for those individuals that step outside of conventional treatment, or simply wish to also utilise a dietary approach in concert with their conventional treatment.

These studies have also pointed out that not everyone responds in the same way. Certainly not everyone has the same load of cancer cells to deal with, but there appears to be more to it than that alone. There are some very large differences in the level of Salvestrol intake required to achieve remission as well as some very large differences in the time taken to achieve remission. One person achieved remission taking as little as 429 Salvestrol points per day, while another took 6,000 Salvestrol points per day to reach the same goal. One person had achieved remission in one month while another took 18 months. All of this tells us that we can't simply pursue an individual's situation from the perspective of statistical averages – each person is unique. We need to gather what information we can from statistical averages, but remain cognizant of the individual differences if one is to have the best chance of recovery. Let's face it, as Steve Hickey and Hilary Roberts pointed out in their book 'Tarnished Gold', if statistical averages were truly representative of us we would all have one testicle and one breast and consequently we would all be quite confused about who we really are!

The rapidity of response of many of these people has driven home the point that upon even the slightest hint of cancer, an individual would be wise to start taking Salvestrols, shifting their diet towards more consumption of organic fruits and vegetables, and making some lifestyle changes that include a bit of daily exercise. There are enough of these individuals responding quickly and dramatically that an early embracing of these changes could spare a person from more aggressive interventions that can come with their own risks and concerns.

In contrast to these rapid responders we have five situations where it took over six months before the individuals reached remission. It is important to remember this as everyone responds differently. For the individual that is not a rapid responder there is still light at the end of the tunnel. Watch for slow and steady progress. So long as you are experiencing slow and steady progress you may simply be one of those that takes longer to respond. Remain vigilant about your diet and supplementation, minimise your exposure to CYP1B1 inhibitors, ensure that you are getting a bit of daily exercise and adequate Salvestrol co-factors and try to remain optimistic about your future health. Don't give up hope – the fellow that took 18 months to achieve remission has now been in remission for close to seven years and is alive a full eight years after his diagnosis!

Phytonutrients rarely have a single mode of action. We have been focused on the mechanism of action brought about by the metabolism of Salvestrols by CYP1B1 but as the people discussed here have informed us there appears to be health benefits above and beyond this anticancer mechanism. The fellow with bladder, kidney and pancreatic cancer reported that his nail fungus cleared up along with his cancer. This report is not unusual to us. We hear of many situations where fungal infections from nail fungus to Candida clear up with Salvestrol use. This is not surprising as Salvestrols are produced in plants as antifungal agents – it appears that they will perform the same function for us. In light of this we should

CONCLUSION

consider fungal infections as a sign that we have a dietary deficiency of Salvestrols and a consequent increase in our risk of developing cancer. An immediate change in diet and commencement of Salvestrol supplementation could turn this around. When we have a fungal infection concurrent with a cancer diagnosis we should increase our daily level of Salvestrol supplementation so that both conditions can be dealt with in a timely fashion.

Another benefit that many of these people report is relief of pain. The cases of breast cancer, colon cancer, anal cancer, CLL, and melanoma all had relief of pain once they started using Salvestrols. Certainly part of the explanation, at least for some of them, would be that once a cancer starts to shrink the pressure on surrounding tissue is diminished with consequent relief of pain. However, we know that some of the Salvestrols also have a powerful anti-inflammatory function and this is also likely to help relieve pain. The cases of colon cancer, CLL and peritoneal cancer all reported a reduction in swelling concurrent with their use of Salvestrols. This too could result from the anti-inflammatory function of various Salvestrols. The woman with ovarian cancer reported that her symptoms associated with osteo-arthritis had all but cleared up. This is another report that is quite common and it too could be due to the anti-inflammatory function of Salvestrols. Of course the fellow with benign prostatic hyperplasia is another report of a health benefit beyond the anticancer activity of Salvestrols. Certainly there may well have been cancer cells that were targeted in his enlarged prostate but it would appear that he benefited from the anti-inflammatory function of Salvestrols as well as perhaps from some benefit that we do not yet understand. These added health benefits are of great interest as they can assist an individual on their road to recovery. We continue to document these reports and hopefully one day we will have the resources to explore these reports through a research and development program aimed at these other benefits.

Perhaps the most significant lesson to be learned is how to remain in remission. The evidence that was gathered during the follow up of these people very, very clearly points out that when addressing a dietary deficiency has brought you through to remission, ensuring that you do not end up with another deficiency will keep you in remission. All of the people that remain in remission continued either taking Salvestrols and/or maintaining a diet rich in organic fruits and vegetables. Remission means that we can no longer detect the presence of cancer – it means that you are somewhere along the curve called the 'Silent Growth of Cancer'. Continued Salvestrol consumption and organic fruit and vegetable consumption will help you remain in the 'Silent Growth' area of the curve and not in the active disease end of the curve.

Certainly these lessons have intensified our efforts at bringing our blood tests to fruition as soon as possible. Reliable and accurate direct measures of the disease will go a long way towards removing uncertainty for both the patient and their practitioner. They will help to point out who is likely to respond very well to a purely nutritional approach to their disease. They will help to point out whether or not an intervention is successful and should be able to do this very soon after commencement of treatment. This alone could spare many people from the risks and concerns of treatments that are not taking them through to remission. Finally, once remission is achieved these tests will be able to provide people with the confidence that they are on the right track to maintain their remission through routine monitoring. We are learning more about this mechanism every day through our research and development of these blood tests and our work with people that have achieved remission through the use of Salvestrols and dietary change. As we analyse more and more samples, our understanding will only improve, and so too will the prospects of those that wish to pursue a nutritional approach to their disease.

The final lesson that we learn from these people predominantly comes from the last two stories – the woman with ovarian cancer and the man that was sent to the hospital to die. Simply put, they tell us what an enormous resource the human mind is in achieving good health. We tend to focus on what can be taken to help achieve remission, to restore life as we would like it to be but we should not forget that our minds can be used to achieve that end and to make the journey a lot more fulfilling while we wait to reach the goal. After all, placebo simply means that good health can be just a thought away, and conversely, nocebo simply means that poor health can be just a thought away. Let's not forget that placebo remains the benchmark against which all treatments are measured – that is, can the treatment outperform the simple thought that I will get better! I realise that it can be difficult when faced with the pain and anguish of a diagnosis to make full use of one's mind to help achieve remission, but it can be done with astonishing results. The good news is that there are many practitioners that have a host of tools at their disposal, such as the auditory technology from the Monroe Institute, to help you make fuller use of your own mind to aid your recovery.

We are always more than the disease we are fighting, more than just a patient, more than the pain we are enduring. A shift in our diet towards organic fruit and vegetable consumption and a shift in our thinking towards good health can turn anguish into joy, despair into optimism and a diagnosis into a path to recovery – and you don't even have to toss your spouse out to do it!

GLOSSARY

Abiraterone acetate	a CYP17 inhibitor, designed by Professor Potter, that is used in last line prostate cancer treatment
adenocarcinoma	a carcinoma that originates in glandular tissue
anaemia	a decrease in the red blood cell count or concentration of hemoglobin
apoptosis	disintegration of damaged or unwanted cells. The bodies mechanism for ridding itself of cells (programmed cell death)
aromatase	aromatase (CYP19) is an enzyme involved in the biosynthesis of estrogens
carcinoma	a malignant cancer that arises from the epithelial cells (cells that line the various structures and organs of our bodies). Carcinoma is the most common type of cancer
carcinogenic	a substance that causes cancer
CYP17	a cytochrome P450 enzyme that is involved in androgen and oestrogen biosynthesis

CYP1B1	a cytochrome P450 enzyme that is intrinsic to cancer cells and not found in healthy tissue
cytochrome P450 enzyme	a superfamily of hemeproteins that are found in animals, plants, fungi and bacteria. They are best known for their drug and toxin metabolism
cystoscopy	viewing the bladder through a lighted, fibre optic system, inserted through the urethra, that transmits the image to the viewer via a lens
dysplastic	evidence of abnormal growth of cells, tissue or organs (dysplasia)
endoscopy	viewing the inside of the body through a lighted tube with a camera at the end
enzyme	a protein in living cells that is capable of producing a biochemical change in other compounds
haematuria	visible blood in the urine
hemoptysis	coughing up blood or bloody sputum
hydrophilic	molecules that have an affinity for and tendency to dissolve in water. Hydrophilic Salvestrols are distributed in the body via the circulatory system

GLOSSARY

lipophilic	molecules that have an affinity for and tendency to dissolve in fats (lipids). Lipophilic Salvestrols are distributed in the body via the lymphatic system and by crossing from cell to cell
liposomal	minute spheres made of phospholipid molecules that contain a water filled cavity that can be used for the delivery of vitamins and other health promoting substances
mutagenic	an agent such as a chemical, ultraviolet light or radioactive element that can alter DNA to cause a mutation
neoplasm	a new and abnormal growth of tissue
neutropenia	an abnormally low number of neutrophils (the most abundant type of white blood cell)
onychomycosis	a very common fungal infection of the finger or toe nails. It accounts for about one third of nail fungal infections
orthomolecular	"orthomolecular medicine describes the practice of preventing and treating disease by providing the body with optimal amounts of substances which are natural to the body." www.orthomed.org
papillary	a projection or growth with a nipple like appearance

paronychia	a fungal or bacterial infection that affects the skin around the finger or toenails
pathogen	an agent that causes disease in another organism
pharmacokinetics	study of the processes of bodily absorption, distribution, metabolism and excretion (ADME) of compounds
phytoalexin	phytoalexins are part of the plant immune system. They are metabolites produced in response to infection by fungus or other pathogen that are inhibitory to the invading pathogen
phytochemistry	a branch of chemistry dealing with the constituents of plants and in particular medicinal plants
phytotherapy	the use of diet and dietary extracts for the maintenance of good health and the recovery of good health
prodrug	a drug or natural compound that relies on enzymatic bioactivation to realise its effect – therapies that would be benign until activated by enzymatic reaction
proteomics	the study of proteins, how and when they are expressed, how they function and how the interact with one another and their involvement in metabolic pathways

GLOSSARY

resection	surgical removal of all or part of a structure, tissue or organ
Salvestrol	natural fungicides found in fruits, vegetables and herbs that are metabolised by the CYP1B1 enzyme in cancer cells to initiate apoptosis in the cancer cell
selectivity	the measure of how well targeted a therapeutic agent is to the cells it is intended to destroy
septicaemia	a life threatening infection characterised by a large amount of bacteria in the blood
squamous cell	squamous cells are epithelial cells that are the main part of the epidermis of the skin
Stilserene	an anticancer agent developed by Professor Potter that is completely targeted to the CYP1B1 enzyme. It is non-toxic to healthy tissue and is metabolised into a toxin by CYP1B1 within the cancer cell
thrombocytopenia	a lower than normal level of platelets in the blood
Zytiga	the brand name for abiraterone acetate the CYP17 inhibitor designed by Gerry Potter

REFERENCES IN THE POPULAR PRESS

Blithe R. February 25, 2013. Cancer and Our Modern Diet. New Zealand Herald, Bite, p.20.

Jacobs, E. January 17, 2013. *Salvestrols: Does Nature Hold the Answer to Cancer?* elynjacobs. http://elynjacobs.wordpress.com/2013/01/17/salvestrols-does-nature-hold-the-answer-to-cancer/

Schaefer, B., Potter G., Wood R., Burke D. Winter 2012/2013. *Nutrition and Cancer: Salvestrol Case Studies.* Health Action Magazine, 16-17.

Ware, W. November/December 2012. *Salvestrols – A natural, targeted approach to preventing and treating cancer.* Integrated Healthcare Practitioners. p. 54-58.

Cheng, J. Fall 2012. Book Review: Salvestrols – Nature's Defence Against Cancer: Linking Diet and Cancer. Health Action Magazine.

Appleton, J. September 2012. *Book review: Salvestrols Nature's Defence Against Cancer.* Channel Magazine, 25, p. 75.

REFERENCES IN THE POPULAR PRESS

Delaney K. July 31, 2012. A Seriously Safe Cancer Medicine That Kills Cancer Not You. Streetarticles.com http://www.streetarticles.com/diseases/a-seriously-safe-cancer-medicine-that-kills-cancer-not-you

Zink M. July 27, 2012. Book Review-Salvestrols, Nature's Defence Against Cancer. herbguide.ca.

http://www.herbguide.ca/members/herbguide/blog/VIEW/00000104/00000112/Book-Review-Salvestrols-Natures-Defence-Against-Cancer.html

Zink M. July 25, 2012. Preventing and Treating Cancer Naturally with Diet. Herbal Collective Magazine. http://herbalcollective.ca/source/2012/07/25/preventing-and-treating-cancer-naturally-with-diet/

Ware W. July/August 2012 edition. *Salvestrol Update.* International Health News. http://www.yourhealthbase.com/ihn229.pdf

Herriot C. June 2012. *Fighting Cancer with Salvestrols.* Common Ground. http://commonground.ca/2012/06/fight-cancer-with-salvestrols/

Henderson B. June 2012. *Salvestrols – Nature's Defence Against Cancer.* CANCER-FREE Newsletter. http://www.beating-cancer-gently.com/161nl.html

Schaefer BA. 2012. *Salvestrols: Nature's Defence Against Cancer, Linking Diet and Cancer.* Clinical Intelligence Corp.

CAHN-Pro Nutrition News and Views, Professional Edition (February 12, 2012). *Nature May Have A Helper To Fight Cancer.*

Schaefer BA. December 2012. *Gerry Potter Honoured for his Development of Abiraterone Acetone, Helping HANS.* http://www.helpinghans.org/show104a2s/Gerry_Potter_Honoured_for_his_Development_of_Abiraterone_Ace

Healy, E. June 2011. *Salvestrols and skin cancer.* CAHN-Pro Nutrition News and Views, Professional Edition, Issue 7. p 1&5.

Schaefer BA, Dooner C, Burke DM, Potter GA, Winter 2010/11 *Nutrition and Cancer: Further Case Studies Involving Salvestrol. Health Action Magazine*, 11-13.

Ware, W. October 2009. *Salvestrol update.* International Health News, Issue 201, p.5. http://www.yourhealthbase.com/ihn_october2009.pdf

Schaefer, B., September 2009 *Abram Hoffer – A Memorial Celebration.* www.hans.org

Schaefer, B., Dooner, C. April 2009 *Does an Apple a Day Keep the Doctor Away?* The Bulletin, WANP.

Wakeman, M. March 2009. *Cancer Cell Science.* Second annual conference: Cancer Prevention and Healing. . DVD available from Health Action Network Society. http://www.hans.org/store/Cancer_Prevention

Dooner, C., Schaefer, B. Spring 2009. *An Apple a Day.* CSNN Holistic Nutrition News.

REFERENCES IN THE POPULAR PRESS

Schaefer BA, Hoon LT, Burke DM, Potter GA, Spring 2008. *Nutrition and Cancer: Salvestrol Case Studies*. Health Action Magazine, 8-9. http://www.hans.org/magazine/278/Nutrition-and-Cancer-Salvestrol-Case-Studies.

Burke, D. March 2008. *Breakthroughs in cancer research from the UK*. First annual conference: Cancer, Natural Approaches for Prevention and Healing. . DVD available from Health Action Network Society. http://www.hans.org/store/Cancer_Prevention

Schaefer, B. Summer 2008. *Salvestrols – Linking Diet and Cancer*. CSNN Holistic Nutrition News.

Ware, W. June 2008. *Salvestrols – A new approach to cancer therapy?* International Health News, Issue 188, p. 1-3. http://www.yourhealthbase.com/archives/ihn188ww.pdf

Peskett, T. Winter 2007. *Organic Wine – A Toast to Disease Prevention*. Health Action Magazine, 27. http://www.hans.org/magazine/389/Organic-Wine

Tan, H. August/September 2007. *Can Food Really be Your Medicine?* Townsend Letter, 116-119.

Schaefer, B. April 2007. *Salvestrols – Linking Diet and Cancer*. Vitality Magazine, 90-91.

Wakeman, M. Spring 2007. *My Voyage Of Discovery Of The Remarkable World Of Salvestrols*. Health Action Magazine, http://www.hans.org/magazine/339/My-Voyage-of-Discovery-from

Schaefer, B., & Tan, H. Mar/Apr 2007. *New Developments in the Science of Salvestrols.* Vista Magazine, 54-55. www.vistamagonline.com

Tan, H. Winter 2007. *Salvestrols: Important New Developments.* Health Action Magazine, 18-19.

Fenn, C. November 2006. *Get a Taste for Salvestrols. Chris Fenn explains why some bitter fruit packs a sweet surprise.* Cycling Plus, 57.

Cox, G. October 2006. *Choices: Organic Cancer-Killers?* Candis, 70-71.

Schaefer, B. Fall 2006. *Salvestrol News.* Health Action Magazine, 30.

Hancock, M. October 2006. *Modern fruits and veggies in a nutritional slump.* Alive Magazine, 36–37.

Schaefer, B. Summer 2006. *Salvestrols vs Cancer: The Story Continues.* Health Action Magazine, 26-27. http://www.hans.org/magazine/355/Salvestrols-vs-Cancer-The-Story-Continues

Underhill, L. July/Aug 2006. *From Red Wine to Bean Sprouts.* Vista Magazine, 20-21. www.vistamagonline.com

Dauncey, G. July 2006. *Winning the Cancer Game.* Common Ground, p. 24. http://www.commonground.ca/iss/0607180/cg180_guy.shtml

REFERENCES IN THE POPULAR PRESS

Atkinson, L. 10:01am 4th July 2006. *You're eating the WRONG fruit and veg!* Daily Mail. http://www.dailymail.co.uk/pages/live/articles/health/dietfitness.html?in_article_id=393956&in_page_id=1798&in_a_source=

Herriot, C. Summer 2006. *The Missing Link.* GardenWise, British Columbia's Gardening Magazine, p. 12.

Schaefer, B., Burke, D. May/June 2006. *Natural Clues to Cancer Intervention.* Vista Magazine, 52-53. www.vistamagonline.com

Schaefer, B. Spring 2006. *Latest Developments in Salvestrol Therapy.* Health Action Magazine, 26-27.

Daniels A. April 2006. *Salvestrols vs Cancer: The Story Continues.* Public Lecture held in Burnaby, B.C. DVD available from Health Action Network Society. http://www.hans.org/store/Cancer_Prevention

Burke, D. March 2006. *Latest Developments in Salvestrol Therapy.* Public Lecture held in Burnaby, B.C. DVD available from Health Action Network Society. http://www.hans.org/store/Cancer_Prevention

Dauncey, G. March 2006. *Organic Food And Cancer.* EcoNews http://www.earthfuture.com/econews/

Herriot, C. March 2006. *The Holy Grail For Cancer.* The Garden Path, www.earthfuture.com/gardenpath

Shannon, K. March 2006. *My Story: From Terminal Cancer to Long Life by Using Salvestrols.*

Schaefer, B. Winter 2006. *Breakthroughs In The Quest To Prevent and Cure Cancer: Professor Potter's BC Lecture Tour.* Health Action Magazine, 28-29.

Burke, D. Winter 2006. *Polymorphisms. What Are They And Why Are They Important?* Health Action Magazine, 26-27, 34.

Kuprowsky, S. Jan/Feb 2006. *Potential Cancer Breakthrough: The New-Found Cancer Killer Inside Certain Vegetables.* Vista Magazine, 20-21. www.vistamagonline.com

Dauncey, G. Jan/Feb 2006. *Cancer, Fruit and Organic Farming: What Are We Doing Wrong?* Vista Magazine, 64-65. www.vistamagonline.com

Schaefer, B. Jan/Feb 2006. *Breakthroughs In The Quest To Cure Cancer.* The Herbal Collective, 29, 31. http://www.herbalcollective.ca

Frketich, K. Winter 2005/2006. *Cancer Research: Lecture Review.* British Columbia Naturopathic Association Bulletin, 12.

Thurnell-Read, J., M.Sc., KFRP. November 2005. *More On Salvestrols, Skin and Tumours.* Life-Work Potential.

Burke, D. Autumn 2005. *Salvestrols – A Natural Defence Against Cancer?* Health Action Magazine, 16-17. http://www.hans.org/magazine/173 Salvestrols-A-Natural-Defence-Against

REFERENCES IN THE POPULAR PRESS

Thurnell-Read, J., M.Sc., KFRP. October 2005. *Eczema, Psoriasis, Parkinson's & Tumours.* Life-Work Potential.

Thurnell-Read, J., M.Sc., KFRP. October 2005. *Skin Problems.* Health and Goodness.

Greene, M. Oct 13th, 2005. *U.K. Doctor Claims Food Enzymes Can Cure Cancer.* The Martlet, Volume 58, Issue 10. http://www.hans.org/newsletters/2005-Fall.pdf

Potter, G. September 2005. *Breakthroughs In The Quest To Prevent and Cure Cancer.* Public Lecture held in Vancouver, B.C. DVD available from Health Action Network Society. http://www.hans.org/store/Cancer_Prevention

Helen Knowles. June 3, 2005. *Will Fruit and Vegetable Plant Salvestrols Save us from Cancers?* Herbsphere. http://www.herbsphere.com/new_page_10.htm

BNN: British Nursing News Online. Thursday, 27 January 2005 16:26. *Fruit and Veg Cure for Cancer.* http://www.bnn-online.co.uk/news_search.asp?-TextChoice=Salvestrol&TextChoice2=&Operator=AND&Year=2005

BBC News UK Edition, Thursday, 27 January, 2005, 11:45 GMT, *Fruit 'Could Provide Cancer Hope'.* http://news.bbc.co.uk/1/hi/england/leicestershire/4211223.stm

The Observer, Sunday January 2, 2005, *Fight Cancer With Food.* http://observer.guardian.co.uk/magazine/story/0,11913,1380969,00.html

Leicester Mercury, September 13, 2003. *Hope in his hands.* P. 11.

Kathryn Senior, 2002. *Molecular Explanation For Cancer-Preventive Properties Of Red Wine.* The Lancet Oncology, Vol. 3, No. 4, 01.

Cancer Research UK, Press Release, Tuesday 26 February 2002. *How A Plant's Anti-Fungal Defence May Protect Against Cancer* http://info.cancer-researchuk.org/pressoffice/pressreleases/2002/february/40684

BBC News Health, Tuesday, 26 February, 2002, 18:11 GMT, *Natural Defence Against Cancer.* http://news.bbc.co.uk/1/hi/health/1841709.stm

Britten, N., & Derbyshire, D. July, 2001. *Tumour-Destroying Drug 'May Be Cure For Cancer'* The Daily Telegraph, 28.

BBC News Health, Friday, 27 July, 2001, 17:09 GMT 18:09 UK, *Cancer Drug Raises Hopes Of Cure.* http://news.bbc.co.uk/1/hi/health/1460757.stm

BIBLIOGRAPHY

American Cancer Society. Cancer Facts and Figures 2012. http://www.cancer.org/acs/groups/content/@epidemiologysurveilance/documents/document/acspc-031941.pdf

Artinyan A, Soriano PA, Prendergast C et al. The anatomic location of pancreatic cancer is a prognostic factor for survival. *HPB (Oxford)* 2008; 10: 371–376.

Attard G, Belldegrun AS, de Bono JS (2005). Selective blockade of androgenic steroid synthesis by novel lyase inhibitors as a therapeutic strategy for treating metastatic prostate cancer. *BJU Int.* **96** (9): 1241–6.

Attard G, Reid AHM, Yap TA, Raynaud F, Dowsett M, Settatree S, Barrett M, Parker C, Martins V, Folkerd E, Clark J, Cooper CS, Kaye SB, Dearnaley D, Lee G, de Bono JS (2008). Phase I Clinical Trial of a Selective Inhibitor of CYP17, Abiraterone Acetate, Confirms That Castration-Resistant Prostate Cancer Commonly Remains Hormone Driven. *Journal of Clinical Oncology* **26**: 4563.

Attard G, Reid A, A'Hern R, Parker C, Oommen N, Folkerd E, Messiou C, Molife L, Maier G, Thompson E, Olmos D, Sinha R, Lee G, Dowsett M, Kaye S, Dearnaley D, Kheoh T, Molina A, and de Bono J (2009). Selective Inhibition of CYP17 With Abiraterone Acetate Is Highly Active in the Treatment of Castration-Resistant Prostate Cancer. *Journal of Clinical Oncology*, **27**(23):3742-8.

BCCA Protocol Summary for Treatment of Hodgkin's Disease with Doxorubicin, Bleomycin, Vinblastine, and Dacarbazine February 1, 2008. http://www.bccancer.bc.ca/NR/rdonlyres/30FDD508-96AC-4555-B682-294EA3635B06/27651/LYABVDProtocol_1Feb08.pdf

Bostwick Laboratories Announces uPM3(TM) Test, First Genetic Test for Prostate Cancer. September 23, 2005. http://www.psa-rising.com/wiredbird/bostwick-labs92303.php

Burke, MD. (2009). The silent growth of cancer and its implications for nutritional protection. *British Naturopathic Journal*, **26**:1, 15-18.

Burke, MD, & Potter, G (2006). Salvestrols ... Natural Plant and Cancer Agents? *British Naturopathic Journal*, **23**:1,10-13.

Campbell, T. Colin, and Campbell, Thomas M. 2006. *The China Study: The Most Comprehensive Study of Nutrition Ever Conducted and the Startling Implications for Diet, Weight Loss and Long-term Health.* BenBella Books.

BIBLIOGRAPHY

Canadian Cancer Society. Breast Cancer Statistics at a Glance. http://www.cancer.ca/Canada-wide/About%20cancer/Cancer%20statistics/Stats%20at%20a%20glance/Breast%20cancer.aspx?sc_lang=en

Canadian Cancer Society. Canadian Cancer Encyclopedia, Colorectal cancer overview. http://info.cancer.ca/cce-ecc/default.aspx?cceid=627&Lang=E&toc=13#Diagnosis

Canadian Cancer Society. Canadian Cancer Encyclopedia. Lung Cancer Overview. http://info.cancer.ca/cce-ecc/default.aspx?cceid=4240&se=yes&Lang=E

Canadian Cancer Society. Canadian Cancer Encyclopedia, Melanoma of the skin. http://info.cancer.ca/cce-ecc/default.aspx?Lang=E&toc=46&cceid=922

Canadian Cancer Society. Canadian Cancer Encyclopedia, Signs and symptoms of colorectal cancer. http://info.cancer.ca/cce-ecc/default.aspx?lf=colorectal&cceid=609&rk=64914833&f-p=file%253a%252f%252fcispublicweb%252fe_html%252f13_4004.html&sqg=2aa29f4d-f9ef-4dc7-b3ff-e4a60aa06365&toc=13

Canadian Cancer Society. Canadian Cancer Encyclopedia, Statistics for Prostate Cancer. http://info.cancer.ca/cce-ecc/default.aspx?toc=41

Canadian Cancer Society. Canadian Cancer Encyclopedia. Survival Statistics for Hodgkin Lymphoma. http://info.cancer.ca/cce-ecc/default.aspx?Lang=E&toc=19

Canadian Cancer Society. Canadian Cancer Encyclopedia, Survival statistics for melanoma. http://info.cancer.ca/cce-ecc/default.aspx?Lang=E&toc=46&cceid=922

Canadian Cancer Society. Canadian Cancer Statistics 2010. Supplementary Figures. http://www.cancer.ca/Canada-wide/About%20cancer/Cancer%20statistics/~/media/CCS/

Canada%20wide/Files%20List/English%20files%20heading/PDF%20-%20Policy%20-%20Canadian%20Cancer%20Statistics%20-%20English/Supplementary%20web %20figures.ashx

Canadian Cancer Society. Colorectal Cancer Statistics at a Glance. http://www.cancer.ca/Canada-wide/About%20cancer/Cancer%20statistics/Stats%20at%20a%20glance/Colorectal%20cancer.aspx?sc_lang=en

Canadian Cancer Society. Prostate Cancer Statistics at a Glance http://www.cancer.ca/Canada-wide/About%20cancer/Cancer%20statistics/Stats%20at%20a%20glance/Prostate%20cancer.aspx?sc_lang=en

BIBLIOGRAPHY

Canadian Cancer Society. Tests for Prostate Cancer http://www.cancer.ca/Canada-wide/Prevention/Getting%20checked/Tests%20for%20prostate%20cancer.aspx?sc_lang=EN*Cancer: New Registrations and Deaths 2000: Revised Edition*. New Zealand Health Information Service, Ministry of Health, Wellington, 2004.

Cancer Research UK. Bladder cancer incidence statistics. http://www.cancerresearchuk.org/cancer-info/cancerstats/types/bladder/incidence/uk-bladder-cancer-incidence-statistics

Cancer Research UK. Bladder cancer statistics and outlook. http://cancerhelp.cancerresearchuk.org/type/bladder-cancer/treatment/bladder-cancer-statistics-and-outlook#general

Cancer Research UK. Breast Cancer Incidence Statistics. http://www.cancerresearchuk.org/cancer-info/cancerstats/types/breast/incidence/

Cancer Research UK. Breast Cancer Survival Statistics. http://www.cancerresearchuk.org/cancer-info/cancerstats/types/breast/survival/

Cancer Research UK. Cancer Incidence for All Cancers Combined. http://www.cancerresearchuk.org/cancer-info/cancerstats/incidence/all-cancers-combined/

Cancer Research UK. Cancer Incidence for Common Cancers. http://info.cancerresearchuk.org/cancerstats/incidence/commoncancers/

Cancer Research UK. Cancer Incidence for Common Cancers. Statistics and outlook for chronic lymphocytic leukaemia (CLL). http://cancerhelp.cancerresearchuk.org/type/cll/treatment/statistics-and-outlook-for-chronic-lymphocytic-leukaemia

Cancer Research UK. Leukaemia survival statistics. http://www.cancerresearchuk.org/cancer-info/cancerstats/types/leukaemia/survival/leukaemia-survival-statistics

Cancer Research UK. Primary Peritoneal Cancer. http://www.cancerresearchuk.org/cancer-help/about-cancer/cancer-questions/primary-peritoneal-carcinoma

Cancer Research UK. Statistics and outlook for chronic lymphocytic leukaemia (CLL). http://cancerhelp.cancerresearchuk.org/type/cll/treatment/statistics-and-outlook-for-chronic-lymphocytic-leukaemia

Carnell DM, Smith RE, Daley FM, et al. (2004) Target Validation of Cytochrome P450 CYP1B1 in Prostate Carcinoma with Protein Expression in Associated Hyperplastic and Premalignant Tissue. *International Journal of Radiation Oncology Biology and Physics* 58: 500-509.

Del Giudice I, Chiaretti S, Tavolaro S, De Propris MS, Maggio R, Mancini F, et al. Spontaneous regression of chronic lymphocytic leukemia: clinical and biologic features of 9 cases. *Blood,* 2009, 114(3):638–46.

du Bois A, Lück HJ, Meier W, et al : A randomized clinical trial of cisplatin/paclitaxel versus carboplatin/paclitaxel as first-line treatment of ovarian cancer. *J Natl Cancer Inst,* 2003; 95: 1320-1329.

Gynecological Cancer Foundation. Understanding Primary Peritoneal Cancer. http://www.wcn.org/downloads/primary_peritoneal_brochure.pdf

Herr HW, Donat SM, Reuter VE: Management of low grade papillary bladder tumors. *J Urol.* 2007; 178(4 Pt 1):1201-5.

Hickey, S., Roberts, H. Tarnished Gold: The Sickness of Evidence Based Medicine. Createspace. 2011.

Jung KW, Park S, Kong HJ, et al: Cancer Statistics in Korea: Incidence, Mortality, Survival and Prevalence in 2008. *Cancer Res Treat.* 2011 March; 43(1): 1–11.

Li NC, & Wakeman M. (October 2009) High-performance liquid chromatography comparison of eight beneficial secondary plant metabolites in the flesh and peel or 15 varieties of apples. *The Pharmaceutical Journal,* supplement Vol. **283**, B40.

Li NC, & Wakeman M. (2009) High-performance liquid chromatography comparison of eight beneficial secondary plant metabolites in the flesh and peel or 15 varieties of apples. *Journal of Pharmacy and Pharmacology,* supplement **1**, A132.

McFadyen MCE, Breeman S, Payne S, et al. Immunohistochemical localization of cytochrome P450 CYP1B1 in breast cancer with monoclonal antibodies specific for CYP1B1. *Journal of Histochemistry and Cytochemistry*, 1999; 47:1457–64.

McKay J, Melvin W, Ahsee A, Ewen S, Greenlee W, Marcus C, Burke M, Murray G (1995) Expression Of Cytochrome-P450 Cyp1b1 In Breast-Cancer *FEBS Letters* **374**(2): 270-272.

Murray GI, McKay JA, Weaver RJ, et al, (1993) Cytochrome P450 expression is a common molecular event in soft tissue sarcomas. *Journal of Pathology*, **171**:49–52.

Murray GI, Melvin WT, Greenlee WF, Burke MD, (2001) Regulation, function, and tissue-specific expression of cytochrome P450 CYP1B1. *Annual Review of Pharmacology and Toxicology*. **41**: 297-316.

Murray GI, Taylor MC, McFadyen MCE, McKay JA, Greenlee WF, Burke MD, Melvin WT (1997) Tumor specific expression of cytochrome P450 CYP 1B1. *Cancer Research*, **57**: 3026-3031.

Neijt JP, Engelholm SA, Tuxen MK, et al: Exploratory phase III study of paclitaxel and cisplatin versus paclitaxel and carboplatin in advanced ovarian cancer. *J Clin Oncol*, 2000; 18: 3084-3092.

BIBLIOGRAPHY

Pan CC, Chang YH, Chen KK, Yu HJ, Sun CH, Ho DM: Prognostic significance of the 2004 WHO/ISUP classification for prediction of recurrence, progression, and cancer-specific mortality of non-muscle-invasive urothelial tumors of the urinary bladder: a clinicopathologic study of 1,515 cases. *Am J Clin Pathol.* 2010; 133(5): 788-95.

Potter GA (2002) The role of CYP 1B1 as a tumour suppressor enzyme. *British Journal of Cancer,* **86** (Suppl 1), S12, 2002.

Potter GA, Burke DM (2006) Salvestrols – Natural Products with Tumour Selective Activity. *Journal of Orthomolecular Medicine,* 21, 1: 34-36.

Product Monograph. Zoladex® 10.8 mg Goserelin/ depot. Luteinizing Hormone – Releasing Hormone Analog (LHRH Analog). February 24, 2009. http://www.astrazeneca.ca/documents/ProductPortfolio/ZOLADEX%20LA_PM_en.pdf

Schaefer, BA. (2013). Case Study: Low grade papillary urothelial carcinoma, kidney cancer and pancreatic cancer. *International Journal of Phytotherapy,* **1**:2, 13.

Schaefer, BA. (2013). Development of Blood Tests for Early Cancer Detection. *International Journal of Phytotherapy,* **1**:2, 7-12.

Schaefer, BA. (2012). Case study follow up: lung cancer. *International Journal of Phytotherapy,* **1**:1, 11.

Schaefer BA. December 2012. *Gerry Potter Honoured for his Development of Abiraterone Acetone,* www.helpingHANS.org.

Schaefer BA. *Salvestrols: Nature's Defence Against Cancer. Linking Diet and Cancer.* Clinical Intelligence Corp., 2012.

Nutrition and Cancer: Further Case Studies Involving Salvestrol. *J Orthomol Med,* 2010; 25, 1: 17-23.

Schaefer BA, Hoon LT, Burke DM, Potter GA: Nutrition and Cancer: Salvestrol case studies. *J Orthomol Med,* 2007; 22: 177-182.

Schaefer, B., Potter G., Wood R., Burke D. Cancer and Related Case Studies Involving Salvestrol and CYP1B1. *J Orthomol Med,* 2012; 27: 131-138.

South Korean National Cancer Center. Cancer Facts and Figures 2011 in the Republic of Korea. http://ncc.re.kr/english/infor/cff.jsp

South Korean National Cancer Center. Cancer Incidence in Korea, 2009. http://ncc.re.kr/english/infor/kccr.jsp

Statistics Canada. Canadian Cancer Statistics 2012. http://www.cancer.ca/Canada-wide/About%20cancer/~/media/CCS/Canada%20wide/Files%20List/English%20files%20heading/PDF%20-%20Policy%20-%20Canadian%20Cancer%20Statistics%20-%20English/Canadian%20Cancer%20Statistics%202012%20-%20English.ashx

Statistics Canada. Cancer, new cases, by selected primary site of cancer, by sex. http://www.statcan.gc.ca/tables-tableaux/sum-som/l01/cst01/hlth61-eng.htm

Vasey PA, Jayson GC, Gordon A, et al: Phase III randomized trial of docetaxel-carboplatin versus paclitaxel-carboplatin as first-line chemotherapy for ovarian carcinoma. *J Natl Cancer Inst*, 2004; 96: 1682-1691.

Vosianov AF, Romanenko AM, Zabarko LB, et al. (1999) Prostatic Intraepithelial Neoplasia and Apoptosis in Benign Prostatic Hyperplasia Before and After the Chernobyl Accident in Ukraine. *Pathology Oncology Research* 5: 28-31.

INDEX

A

abiraterone acetate 160
Abram Hoffer 134, 136, 163
adenocarcinoma 26, 40, 156
Adriamycin 35, 59
albumin 57
Aldara 45, 46
anaemia 84, 156
anal 9, 46, 119
Anthony Daniels xiii, 2, 7, 166
antiandrogen 99
anticancer 160
apoptosis 5, 8, 159
apples 13, 176
aromatase inhibitor 28

B

BBC 168, 169
benign prostatic hyperplasia 103
bicalutamide 99
biotin 32, 98, 113
bladder 9, 14, 15, 16, 17, 19, 21, 25, 104, 117, 132, 157, 174, 176, 177
Blenoxane 59
bleomycin 59
blood 14, 15, 21, 32, 34, 42, 51, 52, 57, 64, 69, 70, 84, 85, 92, 129, 141, 142, 143, 144, 147, 153, 156, 157, 158, 160
BPH 102, 103, 104, 105
brain 3, 27, 93
breast 3, 9, 12, 26, 28, 29, 30, 31, 32, 34, 35, 39, 40, 41, 93, 94, 108, 112, 114, 149, 150, 174, 176
Brian Schaefer 12, 25, 39, 47, 48, 55, 61, 67, 74, 80, 88, 101, 106, 136, 161, 162, 163, 164, 165, 166, 167, 178, 191, 192
bronchoscopy 70

C

CA125 128, 129, 130, 131, 132
Canada ii, 9, 26, 27, 30, 39, 40, 41, 47, 57, 58, 61, 68, 69, 74, 75, 76, 79, 80, 90, 91, 93, 94, 97, 100, 101, 103, 133, 148, 172, 173, 179, 188, 190, 192
cancer 11, 12, 74, 156, 160, 163, 164, 170, 171, 176, 190
candida 84
carboplatin 83, 84, 86, 88, 89, 175, 177, 179
carcinoma 15, 17, 25, 26, 44, 45, 69, 70, 72, 82, 85, 88, 118, 128, 156, 175, 178, 179
CARE Biotechnologies 140
Casodex 99
chemotherapy 31, 35, 36, 37, 38, 58, 59, 60, 64, 70, 77, 81, 83, 84, 85, 88, 108, 110, 112, 113, 129, 130, 149, 179
chronic lymphocytic leukaemia 51, 52, 55, 118, 174, 175
cirrhosis 63, 64, 65, 118
CLL 50, 51, 55, 174, 175
colon 3, 9, 40, 42, 43, 132, 149
colorectal 40, 47, 145, 172
compound 159
CT scan 64, 66, 85
CYP1B1 3, 4, 5, 6, 8, 12, 36, 39, 48, 55, 88, 103, 106, 112, 115, 119, 125, 141, 142, 143, 144, 145, 146, 147, 149, 160, 175, 176, 177, 178
CYP17 2, 4, 11, 156, 160, 170, 171
CYP19 156
cytochrome P450 12, 176, 177

D

dacarbazine 59
Dan Burke xiii, 2, 3, 4, 12, 25, 39, 47, 48, 55, 61, 67, 73, 74, 80, 88, 101, 106, 139, 161, 163, 164, 166, 167, 171, 176, 177, 178
diet 1, 5, 6, 7, 8, 19, 20, 22, 23, 28, 31, 32, 35, 42, 46, 47, 60, 65, 66, 70, 71, 77, 83, 94, 95, 105, 112, 115, 119, 125, 146, 150, 153, 155, 159, 162
dietary change 9, 22, 34, 46, 54, 59, 65, 70,

INDEX

72, 73, 84, 86, 87, 98, 111, 112, 113, 115, 125, 129, 137, 138, 139, 149
dietary deficiency 6, 9, 10, 21, 107, 110, 115, 125, 143, 149, 153
docetaxel 35, 37
doxorubicin 35, 59
DRE 97, 103
DTIC-Dome 59
dysplastic 157

E

endoscopic 58
England 9, 15, 21, 34, 51, 82, 93, 143, 148, 190
enzymatic 159
enzyme 12, 156, 157, 159, 160, 177
epirubicin 17
exercise 1, 19, 22, 32, 34, 65, 95, 98, 115, 125, 150

F

Femera 29, 30
Flomax 104, 105
fruit 165
fungal 7, 8, 16, 158

G

Gerry Potter ix, xiii, 2, 4, 12, 39, 47, 48, 51, 53, 55, 61, 67, 88, 101, 106, 156, 160, 161, 163, 166, 168, 171, 177, 178
goserelin 99

H

haematuria 16, 157
Health Action Magazine 161, 163, 164, 165, 166, 167
Health Action Network Society xiv, 45, 77, 136, 163, 164, 166, 168, 188
hepatitis 63
heritage 8
Hodgkin lymphoma 108, 111, 118
hypothyroidism 31, 33
hysterectomy 83, 85

I

imiquimod 45
impotence 93
infection 16, 84, 144, 158, 159, 160
inhibitor 156
inhibitors 11, 170

Institute of Cancer Research 2
iron 32, 96, 98, 113

K

kidney 15, 17, 19, 20, 21, 23, 25, 98, 117, 118, 178
Korea 9, 62, 63, 67, 148, 176, 179

L

letrozole 28
leuprolide acetate 92, 93
libido 93
lifestyle change 65, 86, 87, 105, 112, 113, 115, 137, 138, 139, 146, 150
liver 9, 27, 62, 63, 64, 65, 66, 118, 149
lung 3, 9, 27, 40, 41, 68, 69, 70, 71, 72, 74, 108, 110, 118, 145, 149, 178
lymph 3, 32, 34, 58, 70, 71, 128

M

magnesium 32, 98, 113
mammogram 29, 34, 36
mass spectrometer 144, 145
meditation 65, 83, 87

melanoma 9, 75, 77, 78, 80, 114, 118, 173
metabolism 159
metabolite 5, 6, 8, 141, 142, 143, 144, 146
metastases 11, 170
Monroe Institute 155, 189
MRI scan 37
mutagenic 158

N

neutropenia 84, 158
New Zealand xv, 9, 14, 15, 25, 148, 161, 173
niacin 32, 65, 98, 113
nocturia 103, 104
nutrition 33, 70, 95, 96, 134

O

oesophagus 3
onychomycosis 16, 20, 158
organic xiii, 7, 32, 36, 70, 71, 77, 105, 112, 115, 119, 125, 150, 153, 155
orthomolecular 158
orthomolecular medicine 158
ovarian 81, 85, 88, 89, 127, 128, 134, 145, 154, 175, 177, 179
Oxford University 190

INDEX

P

paclitaxel 83, 84, 86, 88, 89, 175, 177, 179
pain viii, 17, 28, 31, 33, 34, 35, 42, 43, 46, 52, 53, 58, 64, 69, 77, 78, 79, 84, 130, 154, 155
palliative 134
Panadol 17
pancreas 18, 59
pancreatic 15, 19, 20, 21, 25, 118, 149, 178
papillary 16, 17, 22, 25, 118, 158, 176, 178
Paracetamol 17
paronychia 16, 20, 158
pathogen 158, 159
peritoneal 9, 81, 82, 85, 88, 108, 149, 175
PET scan 71
pharmacokinetics 10, 159
phytoalexin 159
phytoalexins 159
phytochemistry 159
phytotherapy 159
plants 159
probiotic 43, 129
prodrug 5, 6
Prostap 92
proteomic 143, 145, 146
PSA 92, 93, 94, 95, 96, 97, 98, 99, 103

R

radiation 59, 70, 72, 92, 99, 108, 110, 112, 113, 138, 149
radiotherapy 31, 32, 35, 37, 38, 52, 53, 64
rectum 40, 44, 132

remission 9, 10, 15, 20, 21, 22, 23, 24, 27, 29, 31, 33, 34, 38, 41, 43, 44, 46, 47, 50, 51, 54, 58, 60, 63, 66, 69, 72, 73, 76, 79, 82, 87, 92, 94, 95, 96, 97, 99, 100, 105, 107, 110, 112, 114, 115, 117, 118, 125, 128, 132, 138, 141, 148, 149, 150, 153, 154
resection 15, 16, 44, 45, 46, 119, 159
Robbie Wood xiii

S

Salvestrol ii, 9, 10, 15, 19, 20, 21, 22, 25, 27, 28, 29, 30, 31, 32, 33, 34, 35, 39, 41, 42, 43, 44, 46, 47, 48, 51, 53, 54, 55, 58, 59, 60, 61, 63, 64, 65, 66, 67, 69,

70, 71, 72, 73, 74, 76, 77, 78, 80, 82, 83, 87, 88, 91, 93, 95, 96, 97, 98, 99, 100, 101, 103, 104, 105, 106, 107, 108, 109, 110, 111, 112, 114, 115, 117, 118, 119, 125, 127, 128, 129, 141, 142, 143, 149, 150, 153, 159, 161, 162, 163, 165, 166, 168, 178
selectivity 6, 10, 160
selenium 32, 98
septicaemia 16, 160
skin 3, 42, 43, 45, 75, 77, 80, 129, 158, 160, 163, 172
smoking vii
soft tissue sarcomas 12, 177
South Africa 9, 127, 134, 137, 148
squamous cell 44, 45, 69, 70, 72, 160
Stilserene 5, 6, 160
surgery 16, 17, 18, 22, 31, 32, 33, 35, 36, 37, 38, 45, 46, 58, 64, 71, 77, 85, 92, 93, 97, 108, 112, 113, 129, 132, 133, 149

T

Tamoxifen 35
tamsulosin 104
target 160
testis 3
testosterone 2, 3
thrombocytopenia 84, 160
toxin 160
tramadol hydrochloride 17
tuberculosis 64, 65, 118
tumour 12, 177
TURBT 16
Tylenol 31, 58

U

ulcer 52, 53, 64, 65, 118
ultrasound 16, 31, 32, 36, 37, 43
United Kingdom 14, 81
United States 9, 40, 41, 44, 148
University of Victoria 190
uPM3 95, 101, 171
Ural 17
urine 14, 15, 21, 95, 157

V

Velban 59
vinblastine 59
visualisation 83, 87
vitamin C 19, 65, 78, 95, 105, 113, 129
vomiting 42, 83

X

X-ray 29, 34, 36, 92

Y

yoga 32, 34, 66, 115

Z

Zoladex 99, 101, 178
Zytiga 2, 160

FOR MORE INFORMATION

Salvestrols, Nature's Defence Against Cancer.
Linking Diet and Cancer.
Clinical Intelligence Press
Victoria, B.C., Canada
- www.salvestrolbook.com

International Journal of Phytotherapy
- www.ijopt.org

CARE Biotechnologies
Victoria, B.C., Canada
- www.carebiotech.com

Health Action Network Society
214-5589 Byrne Rd
Burnaby BC V5J 3J1
CANADA
- www.hans.org

International Society for Orthomolecular Medicine
16 Florence Avenue
Toronto Ontario
M2N 1E9
CANADA
- www.orthomed.org

Canadian Association of Holistic Nutrition Professionals
CAHN-Pro
150 Consumers Road
Toronto, Ontario M2J 1P9
- www.cahnpro.org

The Monroe Institute
365 Roberts Mountain Road
Faber Virginia, 22938
- www.monroeinstitute.org
- www.monroeinstitute-canada.com

THE AUTHOR

The author was educated in Victoria, B.C., Canada and Oxford, England, obtained a B.Sc., and M.Sc., degree from the University of Victoria and a Doctor of Philosophy (D.Phil.) degree from Oxford University in England (Wolfson College). After these studies were completed he chose to return to Canada. After two years as a research fellow in Ottawa he returned to Victoria to pursue research in the private sector. He currently lives in Victoria with his wife and his two children. A fondness for England continues and he returns to England on a regular basis. He has published and lectured on a broad array of topics including psychometrics, pattern recognition, visual perception, knowledge acquisition, artificial intelligence, laboratory medicine, and cancer research. In 2012 he published his first book 'Salvestrols: Nature's Defence Against Cancer' which is now available in English, Spanish and German. The author serves on the Board of Directors of companies and charities in Canada and England.

CLINICAL INTELLIGENCE PUBLISHING

*Salvestrols: Nature's Defence Against Cancer.
Linking Diet and Cancer*
By Brian A Schaefer

*Salvestroles: La Defensa De La Naturaleza Contra
El Cancer: Vínculos entre dieta y cáncer*
(Spanish Edition)
By Brian A Schaefer

*Salvestrole: Die Antwort der Natur auf Krebs.
Der Zusammenhang zwischen Ernährung und Krebs*
(German Edition)
By Brian A Schaefer

*Les Salvestrols: Une Défense Naturelle Contre le Cancer
Le Rôle Essentiel de l'Alimentation*
(French Version)
By Brian A. Schaefer

*Salvestrolen: Natuurlijke Bescherming Tegen Kanker
Het Verband Tussen Voeding en Kanker*
(Dutch Version)
By Brian A. Schaefer

Clinical Intelligence Corp.
Victoria, B.C., Canada
www.salvestrolbook.com

Printed in Great Britain
by Amazon